Workbook for

PROVIDING HOME CARE
A Textbook for **Home Health Aides**

SECOND EDITION

By Hartman Publishing, Inc.

Credits

MANAGING EDITOR
Susan Alvare

DESIGNER/ILLUSTRATOR
Thaddeus Castillo

COMPOSITION
Thaddeus Castillo/Susan Alvare

PROOFREADER
Suzanne Wegner

Notice to Readers

Though the guidelines and procedures contained in this text are based on consultations with healthcare professionals, they should not be considered absolute recommendations. The instructor and readers should follow employer, local, state, and federal guidelines concerning healthcare practices. These guidelines change, and it is the reader's responsibility to be aware of these changes and of the policies and procedures of her or his healthcare facility. The publisher, author, editors, and reviewers cannot accept any responsibility for errors or omissions or for any consequences from application of the information in this book and make no warranty, expressed or implied, with respect to the contents of the book. The Publisher does not warrant or guarantee any of the products described herein or perform any analysis in connection with any of the product information contained herein.

Copyright Information

© 2004 by Hartman Publishing, Inc.
8529-A Indian School Road, NE
Albuquerque, New Mexico 87112
(505) 291-1274
web: www.**hartman**online.com
e-mail: orders@hartmanonline.com

All rights reserved. No part of this book may be reproduced, in any form or by any means, without permission in writing from the publisher.

ISBN 1-888343-70-2

TABLE OF CONTENTS

Preface 5

Chapter 1
Home Care and the Healthcare System 7

Chapter 2
The Home Health Aide and Care Team 10

Chapter 3
Legal and Ethical Issues 15

Chapter 4
Communication and Cultural Diversity 17

Chapter 5
Infection Control and Standard Precautions 24

Chapter 6
Safety and Body Mechanics 30

Chapter 7
Emergency Care and Disaster Preparation 34

Chapter 8
Physical, Psychological, and Social Health 37

Chapter 9
The Human Body in Health and Disease 40

Chapter 10
Human Development and Aging 48

Chapter 11
Dying, Death and Hospice 53

Chapter 12
Transfers, Ambulation, and Positioning 57

Chapter 13
Personal Care Skills 60

Chapter 14
Core Healthcare Skills 63

Chapter 15
Rehabilitation and Restorative Care 68

Chapter 16
Medications and Technology in Home Care 73

Chapter 17
Clients with Disabilities 76

Chapter 18
Mental Health and Mental Illness 79

Chapter 19
New Mothers, Infants and Children 82

Chapter 20
Common Chronic and Acute Conditions 87

Chapter 21
Clean, Safe and Healthy Environments 100

Chapter 22
Clients' Nutritional Needs 105

Chapter 23
Meal Planning, Shopping, Preparation, and Storage 110

Chapter 24
Managing Time, Energy, and Money 115

Chapter 25
Caring for Yourself and Your Career 117

Procedure Checklists 123-158

4

PREFACE

Welcome to the Workbook! This workbook is designed to help you review what you have learned from reading your textbook. For this reason, the workbook is organized around LEARNING OBJECTIVES, just like the textbook and even your instructor's teaching material.

These learning objectives work as a built-in study guide. After completing the exercises for each learning objective in the workbook, ask yourself if you can DO what that learning objective describes.

If you can, move on to the next learning objective. If you cannot, just go back to the textbook, reread that learning objective, and try again.

We have provided procedure checklists close to the end of the workbook. The answers to the workbook exercises are in your instructor's teaching guide.

Happy Learning!

1

Home Care and the Healthcare System

1. Describe the structure of the healthcare system and describe ways it is changing

Matching.

For each of the following terms, write the letter of the correct definition from the list below.

1. _____ HMOs (health maintenance organizations)
2. _____ Providers
3. _____ Managed care
4. _____ Payers
5. _____ PPOs (preferred provider organizations)
6. _____ Facilities

a. New cost control strategies that are replacing traditional insurance companies
b. People or organizations that provide health care
c. Places where care is delivered or administered
d. A health plan which states that clients must use a particular doctor or group of doctors
e. People or organizations paying for healthcare services
f. A network of providers that contract to provide health services to a group of people

2. Explain Medicare and Medicaid, and list when Medicare recipients may receive home care

True or False.

Mark each statement with either a "T" for true or an "F" for false.

1. _____ To qualify for home health care, Medicare recipients must be unable to leave home.
2. _____ Medicare will pay for any care that the recipient desires.
3. _____ Medicare will only cover people aged 65 or older.
4. _____ Medicaid is a medical assistance program for low-income people.
5. _____ Home health care is never covered by Medicare.
6. _____ Medicare has two parts: hospital insurance and medical insurance.
7. _____ Medicare pays for 100% of all home care.

3. Explain the purpose of and need for home health care

Fill in the Blank.

1. Home care is less _____ than a long hospital or nursing home stay.

2. The growing numbers of _____ and _____ people are also creating a demand for home care services.

3. Home services will be needed to provide continued care and assistance as chronic illnesses progress. For example, _____ is a chronic illness that is infecting more and more people and may require in-home assistance.

4. One of the most important reasons for health care in the home is that most people who are ill or disabled feel more comfortable at _____.

4. List key events in the history of home care services

Multiple Choice.

Circle the letter of the answer that best completes the statement or answers the question.

1. What event happened in 1959 to note the need for home health care?
   a. Homemakers were ordered to war and were therefore unable to help out at home.
   b. A national conference on homemaker services was held.
   c. The Medicare program was created.
   d. A national holiday commemorating homemakers was established.
   e. none of the above

2. When was Medicare created?
   a. 1912
   b. 1996
   c. 1965
   d. 1959
   e. none of the above

3. Why has interest in home health care increased in recent years?
   a. The population of elderly people and people with chronic diseases grew.
   b. Many hospitals closed due to lack of business.
   c. Health care costs increased dramatically.
   d. both a and c
   e. none of the above

4. What is the function of a DRG (diagnostic related group)?
   a. It pairs people with like illnesses together to form a support system.
   b. It offers formal training for people with disabilities to reenter the workplace.
   c. It specifies the treatment cost that Medicare or Medicaid will pay for various diagnoses.
   d. It obtains financial assistance for people with debilitating illnesses.
   e. none of the above

5. Identify the basic methods of payment for home health services

Short Answer.

Identify three of the five basic methods of payment for home health services and write a short description of each.

_____
_____
_____
_____
_____
_____
_____
_____
_____
_____
_____
_____
_____
_____
_____
_____
_____
_____
_____
_____
_____

Name: _____   9

6. Describe a typical home health agency

Labeling.

Fill in the blanks above to complete the diagram of a typical home health agency. Some blanks have already been filled in for you.

7. Explain how working for a home health agency is different from working in other types of facilities

Fill in the Blank.

1. Be aware of personal _____ when you are traveling alone to visit clients.

2. You may have a lot more contact with clients' _____ in the home than you would in a facility.

3. Your supervisor will monitor your work, but you will spend most of your hours working with clients without direct supervision. Thus you must be _____.

4. Good written and verbal _____ skills are important.

5. You will need to be _____ in order to adapt to the changes in environment.

6. In a client's home, you are a _____. Be respectful of the client's property and customs.

2

The Home Health Aide and Care Team

1. Identify the role of each healthcare team member

Matching.

For each of the following terms, write the letter of the correct definition from the list below.

1. ____ Case Manager or Supervisor
2. ____ Home Health Aide (HHA)
3. ____ Medical Social Worker (MSW)
4. ____ Occupational Therapist (OT)
5. ____ Physical Therapist (PT)
6. ____ Physician (MD)
7. ____ Registered Dietitian (RDT)
8. ____ Registered Nurse (RN)
9. ____ Speech Language Pathologist (SLP)

a. Administers therapy in an effort to improve the client's physical status

b. Coordinates, manages, and provides care, as well as supervising HHAs and developing the HHA assignments

c. Diagnoses disease or disability and prescribes treatment

d. Formulates and supervises each client's care plan and makes changes to the care plan when necessary

e. Helps clients get support services, such as counseling

f. Performs delegated tasks, such as taking vital signs, providing personal care, and reporting observations to other care team members

g. Teaches clients and their families about diets to improve health and manage illness

h. Teaches exercises to help the client improve or overcome speech impediments

i. Trains clients to compensate for disabilities during ADLs and other activities

2. Define the client care plan and explain its purpose

True or False.

Mark each statement with either a "T" for true or an "F" for false.

1. ____ The purpose of the client care plan is to give suggestions for care, which the home health aide can customize for each client.

2. ____ Activities that are not listed on the care plan should not be performed without permission from the supervisor.

3. Describe how each team member contributes to the care plan

Short Answer.

List contributions that each of the following team members might make in developing the care plan.

1. Home Health Aide (HHA)

_____

_____

_____

2. Case Manager or Supervisor

_____

_____

_____

Name: _____

3. Physician (MD)
   _____
   _____
   _____
   _____

4. Medical Social Worker (MSW)
   _____
   _____
   _____
   _____

4. Describe the role of the home health aide and explain typical tasks performed

Short Answer.

List and give examples of two ways in which home health aides provide services to their clients.

_____
_____
_____
_____
_____
_____
_____

5. Identify tasks outside the scope of practice for home health aides

True or False.

Mark each statement with either a "T" for true or an "F" for false.

1. _____ Home health aides never administer medications unless they are trained and assigned to do so.

2. _____ Home health aides are trained to perform "invasive" procedures.

3. _____ Home health aides should ignore any requests that are outside of their scope of practice.

4. _____ Home health aides must not accept any request that is not part of their job description or that is not on the assignment sheet.

5. _____ The correct way to deal with unacceptable requests is to explain why the request cannot be met, and report it to the supervisor.

6. _____ Home health aides should not perform procedures that require sterile technique.

7. _____ It is acceptable for home health aides to prescribe certain medications, if they have permission from their supervisor.

8. _____ Home health aides should only inform the client or family of the diagnosis or medical treatment plan if the client asks.

9. _____ Home health aides may perform any task for which they have been trained, even if it is not part of their assignment.

6. List the federal regulations that apply to home health aides

Fill in the Blank.

1. Home health aides must have

   _____
   hours of training and/or pass a

   _____
   before they begin working.

2. Home health aides must have at least 12 hours of

   _____
   every year.

3. It is the responsibility of the

   _____ to
   successfully complete the required in-service training each year.

4. _____ is
   the federal government agency that sets rules and policies to protect workers from hazards on the job.

7. Describe the purpose of the chain of command

Labeling.

Fill in the blanks to complete the diagram of the chain of command.

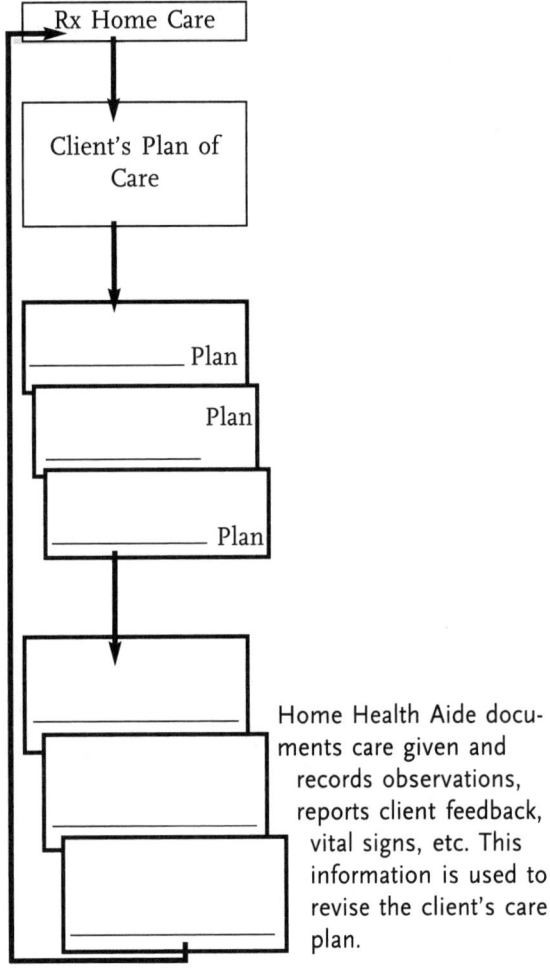

Short Answer

Using the above diagram, answer the following questions.

1. Who orders home care for a client?

   _____
   _____
   _____

2. Who coordinates the plan of care?

   _____
   _____
   _____

3. Who are three care team members who might receive assignments?

   _____
   _____
   _____
   _____

4. What are three types of documentation used for feedback in care planning?

   _____
   _____
   _____
   _____

8. Define policies and procedures and explain why they are important

Short Answer.

List five examples of common policies and procedures at home health agencies.

1. _____
2. _____
3. _____
4. _____
5. _____

9. List examples of a professional relationship with a client and an employer

Read each of the following scenarios and answer the questions.

1. Kathy, a home health aide, wakes up late and decides to skip her morning shower to make up for lost time. She also skips breakfast because she wants to make her first assignment on time. Because she is feeling so rushed, she forgets to respond when her client says, "Good morning." Instead, she complains to her client about her sleepless night, headache, and lack of breakfast.

   Is Kathy behaving in a professional manner?

   _____
   _____
   _____

Name: _____

What should she have done instead?

_____
_____
_____

2. At her next client's home, Kathy asks to use the restroom. She washes her hands carefully when she is finished, and begins to prepare her client's lunch. She listens to her client talk about his grandchildren's visit the day before, and encourages her client to share photographs of the grandchildren. As Kathy is leaving, her client offers her a gift. Kathy politely refuses the gift and explains that it is against her agency's policy.

   List all the examples of Kathy's professional behavior.

   _____
   _____
   _____
   _____
   _____

3. Steve, a home health aide, runs out of time at one client's home and is unable to finish his assignment. When his supervisor finds out, she tells him that he needs to work more efficiently. This makes Steve very upset, and he begins to wonder if his job is worth all the criticism he seems to be getting.

   Is Steve behaving in professionally?

   What should he have done instead?

   _____
   _____
   _____
   _____

4. At his next meeting with his supervisor, Steve explains why he was unable to finish his assignment and asks his supervisor for suggestions. She shows him how to organize his time more efficiently. After asking several more questions, Steve feels that he now understands how to work more effectively. Being able to communicate in a positive way with his supervisor improves Steve's attitude about his job.

   List all the examples of Steve's professional behavior.

   _____
   _____
   _____
   _____
   _____
   _____

10. Demonstrate how to organize care assignments

Short Answer.

1. Discuss why it is important to organize your work.

   _____
   _____
   _____
   _____
   _____

2. Why should you include the client in planning your schedule?

   _____
   _____
   _____
   _____
   _____

11. Demonstrate good personal grooming habits

Word Search.

```
h j e w e l r y b w t y s
p c u k n b m q y n g l x
o i e o z y o d a g e r g
z e h m p n n r a t h a h
s m k z t f o b p r j s g
e u h n e d w i b t q h n
h f s b o e e d g u r i i
t r m e x k u x t d b m r
o e d r e t l o s o v g e
l p i w u m x t y r t n w
c a b a t h i n g y j w o
h e j r g n i m o o r g h
r o l k h w c s u l j y s
```

Complete each of the following sentences and then find the answers in the word search.

1. Good _____ makes you feel great and others feel good about you.

2. _____ or _____ daily are important parts of good grooming.

3. Wash and iron your _____ regularly.

4. Do not wear clothes that are too _____.

5. Long _____ should be tied back in a bun or ponytail.

6. Use _____ or anti-perspirant every day.

7. Do not wear _____ as some clients may not be tolerant of some odors.

8. Never wear _____ that is too large or gets in the way.

12. Identify personal qualities a home health aide must have

Short Answer.

From this learning objective in the textbook, pick three qualities that you believe you can improve in yourself, and describe how you will improve on these qualities.

1. _____

2. _____

3. _____

13. Identify an employer's responsibilities

Short Answer.

List and describe four responsibilities of the employer to the home health aide.

1. _____

2. _____

3. _____

4. _____

3

Legal and Ethical Issues

1. List examples of legal and ethical behavior

Short Answer.

Read each of the following scenarios and answer the questions.

1. Sarah, a home health aide, is out shopping with her friends. One of them asks her if she likes her job, and she responds enthusiastically. She proceeds to relate to them that her client, Mrs. Daly, has Alzheimer's disease and has to be reminded of her name several times a day, as she is apt to forget it.

    Did Sarah behave in a legal and ethical manner? Why or why not?

    _____

    _____

    _____

    _____

2. Caroyl, a home health aide, finishes her duties for the day early. Her client, Mr. Leach, tells her how pleased he is with her work. He says that she is the first aide that has made him feel so comfortable and well taken care of. He gives her a little box of candy and says it is for all the hard work she has done. Caroyl initially refuses, but after he insists, she takes it from him, thanking him.

    Did Caroyl behave in a legal and ethical manner? Why or why not?

    _____

    _____

    _____

    _____

    _____

3. Charlie, a home health aide, has been working for Mrs. Castillo for almost a year. Her family is visiting from out-of-state and Charlie meets her daughter, Susan, for the first time. During the course of conversation, Susan asks Charlie to come have a drink with her so that they can talk about her mother's case in a more relaxed environment. Charlie tells her that he can go out for a short while. They arrange to meet.

    Did Charlie behave in a legal and ethical manner? Why or why not?

    _____

    _____

    _____

    _____

    _____

    _____

2. List examples of clients' rights and explain why they are important

True or False.

Mark each statement with either a "T" for true or an "F" for false.

1. _____ It is okay to abuse a client psychologically, but never verbally or physically.

2. _____ If a home health aide suspects that a client is being abused, he should keep quiet, in order to not get anyone angry at him.

3. _____ Clients have the right to participate in their care planning.

4. _____ Clients should only be informed of obstacles or barriers to their care if they are life-threatening.

5. _____ Neglect is the failure of a caregiver to take proper care of a person.

6. _____ Clients should never know what the agency expects to happen as a result of their care.

3. List examples of behavior supporting and promoting clients' rights

Multiple Choice.

Circle the letter of the answer that best completes the statement.

1. When performing a procedure on your client, you should:
   a. try to distract them so they won't know what you're doing
   b. explain the procedure fully before performing it
   c. wait until they're sleeping before you start the procedure
   d. always notify the physician first
   e. none of the above

2. If a client refuses to take a bath, you should:
   a. offer them a prize if they will take the bath
   b. respect their wishes, but report it to your supervisor
   c. tell them you are going to leave if they don't comply
   d. force them to take the bath
   e. none of the above

3. If another home care aide asks you about your client's care plan, you should:
   a. explain that you can't talk or gossip about your client
   b. tell them about the care plan
   c. say "I'll tell if you go first."
   d. tell them only about your client's diet/nutrition plan but nothing else
   e. none of the above

4. If you suspect your client is being abused, you should:
   a. open his mail and look through his belongings to find any clues
   b. call your closest friends and ask their advice
   c. report it to your supervisor immediately
   d. check with their relatives first
   e. none of the above

4. Explain HIPAA and list ways to protect clients' confidentiality

Short Answer.

1. What can happen to healthcare facilities and their employees if they do not follow HIPAA?

   _____
   _____
   _____
   _____
   _____

2. What can you say to a person who is not part of the care team when they ask you about your client?

   _____
   _____
   _____
   _____
   _____

4

Communication and Cultural Diversity

1. Define communication

Short Answer.

1. List the three basic steps of communication.

   _____
   _____
   _____
   _____
   _____
   _____

2. Why is feedback an important part of communication?

   _____
   _____
   _____
   _____
   _____
   _____
   _____

3. With whom must home health aides be able to communicate?

   _____
   _____
   _____
   _____
   _____
   _____

2. Explain verbal and nonverbal communication

Multiple Choice.

Circle the letter of the answer that best completes the statement or answers the question.

1. Which of the following is an example of nonverbal communication?
   a. asking for a glass of water
   b. pointing to a glass of water

2. Types of verbal communication include:
   a. writing
   b. nodding your head
   c. speaking
   d. both a and c
   e. all of the above

3. Types of nonverbal communication include:
   a. speaking
   b. facial expressions
   c. the way in which you say something
   d. both b and c
   e. none of the above

4. Which of the following is an example of a confusing or conflicting message (saying one thing and meaning another)?
   a. Mr. Carter smiles happily and tells you he is excited because his daughter is coming to visit.
   b. Mrs. Sanchez looks like she is in pain. When you ask her about it, she tells you that her back has been bothering her.
   c. Ms. Jones agrees with you when you say it is a nice day, but she looks angry.
   d. Mr. Wilson won't watch his favorite TV show. He says he feels a little depressed.
   e. none of the above

5. In the previous question, how would you clarify the confusing or conflicting message?
   a. state what you have observed and ask if the observation is correct
   b. ignore the conflicting message and accept what the person has told you
   c. ask the person to repeat what he or she has just said
   d. tell the person that you know they are not telling the truth
   e. none of the above

3. Identify barriers to communication

Crossword.

Across

2. Your client or the family may not understand _____ terminology.
4. Avoid using _____ words that are unprofessional.
6. Be _____ with a client who is difficult to understand
8. Do not give medical _____ to the client or family.
10. Keep in mind that _____ language is also part of your message, and be aware of it.
11. Make sure you speak clearly, especially if your client is hard of _____.

Down

1. Ask _____ questions to get more information from the client.
3. Yes or no answers bring the _____ to an end.
5. _____ are phrases that don't really mean anything.
7. Do not offer your personal _____ to the client or family.
9. Avoid asking _____ when your client makes a statement.

4. List ways to make communication accurate and complete

Short Answer.

List six techniques that can help you send and receive clear, complete messages:

1. _____
2. _____
3. _____
4. _____
5. _____
6. _____

Name: _____

5. Describe the difference between facts and opinions

Fact or Opinion.

For each statement, decide whether it is an example of a fact or an opinion. Write "F" for fact or "O" for opinion in the space provided.

1. _____ It's better to take your bath before you eat.
2. _____ You'll get depressed if you stay in your pajamas all day.
3. _____ It's not fair for you to give me a present.
4. _____ My agency says I cannot accept a gift.
5. _____ Your care plan calls for snacks between meals.
6. _____ Mr. Ford drinks more coffee than is good for him.
7. _____ Mr. Ford drinks three cups of coffee every morning.
8. _____ Mrs. Myers needs assistance to stand up.
9. _____ Mrs. Myers looks like she is in a lot of pain.

6. Explain how to develop effective interpersonal relationships

True or False.

For each of the following statements, write "T" if the suggestion will help develop good relationships with clients, and write "F" if it will not.

1. _____ Put yourself in other people's shoes.
2. _____ If a subject makes you feel uncomfortable, change the subject.
3. _____ Lean forward in your chair when listening to someone.
4. _____ Do not talk down to your client.
5. _____ Requests that you cannot honor should be ignored.
6. _____ Tell clients that you know how they feel.
7. _____ Approach the person who is talking.

7. Describe basic medical terminology and approved abbreviations

Matching.

For each of the following abbreviations, write the letter of the correct term from the list below.

1. _____ ac
2. _____ amb
3. _____ B.M.
4. _____ C
5. _____ c/o
6. _____ CPR
7. _____ F
8. _____ ft
9. _____ GI
10. _____ hs
11. _____ I&O
12. _____ NPO
13. _____ OOB
14. _____ pc
15. _____ qid
16. _____ R
17. _____ ROM
18. _____ SOB
19. _____ VS
20. _____ w/c

a. Fahrenheit degree
b. hours sleep
c. after meals
d. nothing by mouth
e. bowel movement

f. cardiopulmonary resuscitation
g. complains of
h. range of motion
i. respirations
j. vital signs
k. shortness of breath
l. before meals
m. foot
n. wheelchair
o. four times a day
p. intake and output
q. Celsius degree
r. out of bed
s. gastrointestinal
t. ambulate

8. Explain how to give and receive an accurate oral report of a client's status

True or False.

Mark each statement with either a "T" for true or an "F" for false.

1. _____ Oral reports are used to report something immediately to the supervisor.
2. _____ Oral reports are never used to discuss the home health aide's observations of the client.
3. _____ Oral reports are only opinions.
4. _____ Before giving an oral report, make notes to help you remember the basic information.
5. _____ It is not necessary to document an oral report.
6. _____ Do not take notes during a supervisor's oral report, since this can be a distraction.
7. _____ Restate what you have been told to make sure you understand it.
8. _____ After giving an oral report, you must make a written report later.
9. _____ Anything that endangers the client should be reported at the next staff meeting.
10. _____ You may use oral reports from other home health aides to help you with a new client.

9. Demonstrate how to report and document factual observations in written or oral form

Labeling.

Looking at the diagram, list examples of observations using each sense.

Smell: _____
Sight: _____
Hearing: _____
Touch: _____

For each of the following, decide whether it is an objective observation (you can see, hear, smell, or touch it) or subjective observation (the client must tell you about it). Write "O" for objective and "S" for subjective.

1. _____ Skin rash
2. _____ Crying
3. _____ Rapid pulse
4. _____ Headache
5. _____ Nausea

Name: _____

6. _____ Vomiting
7. _____ Swelling
8. _____ Cloudy urine

10. Explain why documentation is important and describe how to document visit records and incident reports

Short Answer.

List three reasons why it is essential that you maintain current documentation for your clients.

1. _____
   _____
   _____
   _____
   _____

2. _____
   _____
   _____
   _____
   _____

3. _____
   _____
   _____
   _____
   _____

True or False.

Mark each statement with either a "T" for true or an "F" for false.

1. _____ A medical chart is a legal document.
2. _____ Medical charts are not proof that care was given to a client.
3. _____ The information in a medical chart is always confidential.
4. _____ Failing to document visits and activities will not cause any harm to the client.
5. _____ If you didn't document it, legally you did not do it.
6. _____ Visit notes should be written at the end of the day when there is more time to write.
7. _____ The purpose of visit notes is to serve as a record of the home health aide's visit and the care provided.
8. _____ To help you present your thoughts as briefly and clearly as possible, you should simply write and not spend a lot of time initially thinking about what you are going to write.
9. _____ Include your own thoughts and opinions about the visit in the visit notes.
10. _____ If you make a mistake, erase the mistake or use correction fluid.
11. _____ After completing each day's visit notes, sign your full name, your title, and the date.
12. _____ Incidents must be reported before leaving the client's home.
13. _____ Do not report an incident that makes you feel uncomfortable unless you think it might be a direct threat to you.
14. _____ If your client breaks something, you should file an incident report.
15. _____ Incident reports are meant to protect you, the client, and your agency.

11. Demonstrate ability to use verbal and written information to assist with the care plan

Short Answer.

1. If you are not sure what is important to mention in a care plan meeting, you should:

   _____
   _____
   _____
   _____
   _____
   _____
   _____

2. Why do you think your accurate reporting is so important to the other members of the care team?

_____
_____
_____
_____

12. Demonstrate effective communication on the telephone

Read the following telephone conversations and think about how the home health aide could have better presented herself on the phone.

Example #1 Leaving a message for the supervisor

Hi, who's this?

Could you get Ms. Crier on the phone, please? I need to talk to her.

She's not there? Do you know where she is? I really have to talk to her right now. My client forgot to take her pill this morning and now she wants to take two and I don't know if that's okay or not, so that's why I need to talk to Ms. Crier.

Okay, well tell her Ella called and have her call me back. Ella. Ella Ferguson. I should be on the schedule.

The number? I don't remember what it is. Let me ask the client.

Okay, the number is 873-9042. I don't know how much longer I'll be here, but have her call me as soon as possible. Bye.

1. What did the home health aide do wrong in this phone conversation?

_____
_____
_____
_____

Example #2 Answering calls for the client

Hello? Mrs. Lee? No, she can't come to the phone right now. She's in the bathroom. Who's calling?

And your number?

Can I tell her what this is about?

Okay. I'll give her the message. Goodbye.

2. What did the home health aide do wrong in this phone conversation?

_____
_____
_____
_____
_____
_____
_____
_____

13. Describe cultural diversity and religious differences

Fill in the Blank.

For each sentence below, write down which religion it refers to using the words below. Some words may be used more than once.

    Buddhism   Hinduism
    Christianity   Islam
    Confucianism Judaism

1. Worship at mosques.

_____

2. Practice religion mostly in China and Japan.

_____

3. Take communion as a symbol of Christ's sacrifice.

_____

Name: _____

4. Believe that Allah (God) wants men to follow the teachings of the prophet Mohammed in the Koran.
   _____

5. Religious leaders may be called priests, ministers, pastors, or deacons.
   _____

6. Believe that God gave them laws through Moses and in the Bible, and that these laws should order their lives.
   _____

7. Pray five times a day facing Mecca.
   _____

8. This religion started in Asia.
   _____

9. May not do certain things, such as work or drive, on the Sabbath.
   _____

10. Believe Jesus Christ was the son of God and that he died so their sins would be forgiven.
    _____

11. Practice their religion in India and elsewhere.
    _____

12. Religious leaders are called rabbis.
    _____

14. List examples of cultural and religious differences

Short Answer.

List three dietary restrictions due to religious beliefs.

1. _____
2. _____
3. _____

15. List ways of coping with combative behavior

Fill in the Blank.

1. Clients may sometimes display _____ behavior.

2. This behavior may be the result of _____ affecting the brain, an expression of _____, or part of someone's _____.

3. Do not take such behavior _____.

4. Always _____ combative behavior to your supervisor and be sure to _____ it.

5. It is important for other members of the care team to be _____ of this behavior.

16. List ways of coping with inappropriate behavior

Short Answer.

1. List three examples of inappropriate behavior from the client.
   _____
   _____
   _____
   _____
   _____
   _____
   _____
   _____

2. For each example listed in #1, write down how you should respond to the inappropriate behavior.
   _____
   _____
   _____
   _____
   _____
   _____
   _____

5

Infection Control and Standard Precautions

1. Define asepsis and explain the chain of infection

Multiple Choice.

Circle the letter of the answer that best completes the statement or answers the question.

1. The following are necessary links in the chain of infection. By wearing gloves, which link is broken, thus preventing the spread of disease?
   a. reservoir (place where the pathogen lives and grows)
   b. mode of transmission (a way for the disease to spread)
   c. susceptible host (person who is likely to get the disease)
   d. none of the above

2. The following are necessary links in the chain of infection. By getting a vaccination shot for Hepatitis B, which link will be affected and thus prevent you from getting Hepatitis B?
   a. reservoir (place where the pathogen lives and grows)
   b. mode of transmission (a way for the disease to spread)
   c. susceptible host (person who is likely to get the disease)
   d. none of the above

3. The single most important thing you can do to prevent the spread of disease is to:
   a. carry dirty linen close to your uniform
   b. never change your gloves
   c. remove gloves before cleaning spills
   d. wash your hands

2. Identify when to wash hands

True or False.

Mark each statement with either a "T" for true or an "F" for false.

1. _____ You should wash your hands every time you remove your gloves or any type of PPE.

2. _____ You should only wash your hands on arrival at a client's house, never before you leave it.

3. _____ You don't have to wash your hands if you come into contact with saliva.

4. _____ When working in the kitchen, only wash your hands if you're preparing a meat dish.

5. _____ You should wash your hands after using the restroom.

3. Identify when to wear gloves

Mark an "X" next to the tasks that require you to wear gloves.

1. _____ handling body fluids
2. _____ hanging the laundry
3. _____ potentially touching blood
4. _____ brushing the client's hair
5. _____ performing or assisting with perineal care
6. _____ washing vegetables
7. _____ putting clean sheets on an unoccupied bed
8. _____ performing or assisting with mouth care
9. _____ shaving a client

Name: _____

4. Identify when to use personal protective equipment (PPE)

Word Search.

Complete each of the following sentences and find your answers in the word search.

1. A _____ should be worn when caring for clients with respiratory illnesses.

2. Eye _____ are worn when splashing of body _____ or _____ could occur.

3. If there is a chance you could come into contact with _____ membranes or open wounds, you should wear _____.

4. A mask, glove, eye shield, and _____ are all examples of PPE.

t	y	v	f	q	n	m	h	q	i	e	f	c	s
j	x	t	i	f	z	z	u	s	y	w	z	u	v
b	n	f	r	u	h	s	a	e	t	i	o	l	p
k	w	s	m	u	u	r	d	p	t	c	g	q	a
u	d	f	w	q	w	k	j	l	u	d	m	m	t
o	s	l	x	d	n	w	k	m	e	s	t	m	z
y	c	m	c	l	i	n	y	q	i	i	r	k	p
d	x	p	t	t	v	u	w	j	q	i	h	g	p
o	w	q	t	c	a	u	s	o	i	k	s	s	e
o	a	q	k	k	x	y	k	o	g	h	n	r	d
l	o	s	w	q	b	q	p	c	z	e	j	w	a
b	a	q	c	c	c	j	b	c	p	i	d	k	l
m	a	n	y	w	w	y	f	s	j	o	e	o	u
k	i	f	z	f	l	u	i	d	s	v	g	c	l

5. Explain how to handle spills

Short Answer.

Read the following scenario and answer the questions below.

Eddie, a home health aide, takes a urine sample from his client, Mr. Velasquez. When he finishes, he accidentally knocks the container onto the linoleum floor. Some of the urine spills out before he can get to it. Eddie quickly grabs a sponge and begins to wipe up the spill. When he is finished, he finds the mop, puts dishwashing soap into a bucket, and cleans the area again. When he is done mopping, he washes his hands.

Did Eddie follow the proper spill-handling procedure?

_____

If not, what should Eddie have done?

_____
_____
_____
_____
_____
_____
_____
_____
_____
_____
_____
_____
_____

6. Explain and follow Standard Precautions

True or False.

Mark each statement with either a "T" for true or an "F" for false.

1. _____ Standard Precautions means treating all blood, body fluids, non-intact skin, and mucous membranes as if they were infected with an infectious disease.

2. _____ Standard Precautions relate to all body fluids except saliva.

3. _____ You can usually tell if someone is infectious by looking at them.

4. _____ The Centers for Disease Control and Prevention defined Standard Precautions.

5. _____ You should wash your hands before putting on gloves.

6. _____ It is okay for you to handle your clients' needles or syringes.

7. _____ Giving mouth care will require you to wear gloves.

8. _____ It's a good idea to wear a mask and protective goggles if you're emptying a bedpan.

9. _____ When cleaning a urinal, you do not need to wear gloves.

Multiple Choice.

Circle the letter of the answer that best completes the statement or answers the question.

10. Standard Precautions should be practiced:
    a. only on people who look like they have a bloodborne disease
    b. on every single person in your care
    c. only on people who request that you follow them
    d. none of the above

11. Standard Precautions include the following measures:
    a. Washing your hands before putting on and after removing gloves
    b. Wearing gloves if there is a possibility you will come into contact with blood, body fluids, mucous membranes, or broken skin
    c. Touching body fluids with your bare hands
    d. a and b

12. Which of the following is true for Transmission-Based Precautions?
    a. You do not need to practice Standard Precautions if you practice Transmission-Based Precautions.
    b. They are exactly the same as Standard Precautions.
    c. They are practiced in addition to Standard Precautions.
    d. none of the above

7. Explain guidelines of care for clients with infectious diseases

True or False.

Mark each statement with either a "T" for true or an "F" for false.

1. _____ If you are using isolation precautions, you do not use Standard Precautions.

2. _____ Family members can use the same dishes as the person who is in isolation.

3. _____ A client in contact or airborne isolation should have a separate bathroom to use.

4. _____ You should wear disposable gloves when handling soiled laundry.

5. _____ Bleach solutions can be used to clean up spills of blood or body fluids and to disinfect surfaces that may have been contaminated.

6. _____ When following isolation procedures, disposable dishes and utensils do not have to be discarded in any particular way.

8. Explain sterilization and disinfection

Short Answer.

1. How does wet heat disinfect? How does dry heat disinfect?

   _____
   _____
   _____
   _____

2. What is the difference between sterilization and disinfection?

   _____
   _____
   _____
   _____

Name: _____

9. Explain how bloodborne diseases are transmitted

Short Answer.

1. Explain how bloodborne diseases can be transmitted.

   _____
   _____
   _____
   _____
   _____
   _____
   _____
   _____
   _____
   _____
   _____

2. Name three methods of preventing transmission of bloodborne diseases.

   _____
   _____
   _____
   _____
   _____
   _____
   _____
   _____
   _____
   _____
   _____

10. Explain the basic facts regarding HIV and hepatitis infection

Fill in the Blank.

1. Hepatitis refers to swelling of the _____ caused by infection.

2. The major bloodborne diseases in the United States today are _____ and _____.

3. There is no vaccine for hepatitis _____.

4. After a number of years, a person with HIV usually develops _____.

5. When people are infected with HIV, the disease weakens their _____ system so that their bodies cannot effectively fight infections.

6. Your employer must offer you a free vaccine to protect you from hepatitis _____.

7. The risk of acquiring _____ is greater than the risk of acquiring _____.

8. People with AIDS can lose all ability to fight _____ and can die from illnesses that a healthy body could handle.

9. Hepatitis _____ and _____ are bloodborne diseases that can cause death.

11. Identify high risk behaviors that allow the spread of HIV/AIDS and HBV

True or False.

Mark each statement with either a "T" for true or an "F" for false.

1. _____ You are at a high risk for HIV/AIDS if you hug an HIV positive person.

2. _____ You can protect against the spread of HIV/AIDS by never sharing used drug needles.

3. _____ Abstinence means having sex with only one person.

28

Name: _____

4. _____ You are at a high risk for HIV/AIDS if you are having unprotected sex.

5. _____ It may take six months after coming into contact with the virus for an HIV test to show positive.

6. _____ Pregnant women should not get tested for HIV.

7. _____ Having sexual contact with many partners puts you at a high risk for HIV/AIDS.

12. Demonstrate knowledge of the legal aspects of AIDS, including testing

Short Answer.

1. If you had just met someone and they told you they had AIDS, how would you feel?

   _____
   _____
   _____
   _____
   _____
   _____
   _____

2. What are your thoughts on the right to privacy regarding health status?

   _____
   _____
   _____
   _____
   _____
   _____
   _____

13. Identify community resources and services available to clients with HIV/AIDS

Word Search.

Complete each of the following sentences and find your answers in the word search.

1. There are many resources available for clients who have _____ or _____.

2. Meal services, _____, and access to experimental _____ are all examples of _____ available to clients with HIV/AIDS.

3. You can check the phone book or the internet for _____ available in your area.

4. A member of the care team or a _____ may be able to _____ services for clients with HIV/AIDS.

n	g	t	j	g	n	i	l	e	s	n	u	o	c
e	e	f	i	c	g	s	e	c	i	v	r	e	s
z	n	t	k	s	d	o	c	b	z	d	z	s	r
z	k	b	a	g	r	u	p	l	l	g	g	e	v
p	a	q	i	n	y	l	x	e	j	u	k	l	o
s	p	e	g	t	i	s	m	h	r	r	y	j	o
e	n	z	q	s	e	d	p	d	o	c	i	m	s
c	g	w	w	f	i	o	r	w	f	e	g	l	x
r	u	g	w	v	s	a	l	o	q	h	s	d	u
u	a	u	g	k	i	a	o	u	o	o	s	y	z
o	b	b	g	d	i	w	z	v	s	c	u	c	o
s	h	w	s	c	l	j	g	w	g	n	h	v	x
e	m	l	o	c	k	x	j	x	s	r	a	i	s
r	w	s	q	q	z	b	q	m	f	l	h	e	v
c	o	m	m	u	n	i	t	y	r	c	i	s	m

Name: _____

14. Explain tuberculosis and list infection control guidelines

Multiple Choice.

Circle the letter of the answer that best completes the statement.

1. Tuberculosis may be transmitted:
   a. by coughing
   b. by dancing
   c. through the air
   d. both a and c
   e. none of the above

2. Tuberculosis is:
   a. a bloodborne disease
   b. an airborne disease
   c. an infectious disease
   d. both b and c
   e. both a and c

3. Someone with a TB infection:
   a. shows symptoms
   b. falls into a coma almost immediately
   c. cannot infect others
   d. all of the above
   e. none of the above

4. A person with active TB:
   a. can spread it to others
   b. does not show symptoms
   c. cannot eat whole foods
   d. all of the above
   e. none of the above

5. TB disease is more likely to develop in people:
   a. who live near the mountains
   b. whose relatives had it when they were kids
   c. whose immune systems are weakened
   d. all of the above
   e. none of the above

6. One major factor in the spread of TB is:
   a. failure to take all the medication prescribed
   b. following Standard Precautions
   c. wearing a gown and mask during client care
   d. following isolation procedures if indicated in the care plan

15. Explain the importance of reporting a possible exposure to an airborne or bloodborne disease

Short Answer.

How do you report possible exposure to an airborne or bloodborne disease?

_____
_____
_____
_____
_____
_____
_____
_____
_____
_____

16. Explain the terms MRSA and VRE

True or False.

Mark each statement with either a "T" for true or an "F" for false.

1. _____ MRSA is spread by direct physical contact.

2. _____ MRSA is not spread through the air.

3. _____ If VRE is established, it is relatively easy to get rid of it.

4. _____ MRSA is spread through indirect contact by touching objects.

5. _____ Handwashing will not help control the spread of MRSA.

6
Safety and Body Mechanics

1. Explain the principles of body mechanics

Labeling.

Complete the illustration by labeling each part with the words listed below.

alignment
base of support
center of gravity
fulcrum
lever

1. _____
2. _____
3. _____
4. _____
5. _____

2. Apply principles of body mechanics to your daily activities

A.   B.

Short Answer.

1. Which picture shows the correct way to lift objects? Why is it correct?
   _____
   _____
   _____
   _____
   _____
   _____

Fill in the Blank.

2. When you stand up, _____ with your strong hip and thigh muscles to raise your body and the object together.

3. Bend your _____ to lower yourself, rather than bending from the _____.

4. Get _____ whenever possible for lifting or assisting clients.

5. Hold objects _____ to you when you are lifting or carrying them.

6. Avoid _____ at the waist. Instead, turn your whole body.

7. If you are making an adjustable bed, adjust the _____ to a safe working level.

8. Never try to _____ a falling client.

9. Spread your feet _____

Name: _____   31

apart and bend your knees when lifting an object from the floor.

10. _____, _____, or _____ objects rather than lifting them.

3. List ways to adapt the home to principles of good body mechanics

Multiple Choice.

Circle the letter of the answer that best completes the statement.

1. If you cannot reach an object on a high shelf, you should
   a. stand on tiptoes to reach it
   b. use a stepstool
   c. climb on a counter or lower shelf
   d. all of the above
   e. none of the above

2. When sitting for long periods of time, you should not cross your legs because
   a. it disrupts the alignment of your body
   b. it can cause discomfort
   c. it is unprofessional
   d. both a and b
   e. none of the above

3. To be more comfortable doing tasks that require standing for long periods of time, you can
   a. sit down every five minutes
   b. stand on one foot
   c. place one foot on a footrest
   d. all of the above
   e. none of the above

4. Frequently-used tools and supplies should be placed
   a. on shelves or counters to reduce the need for bending
   b. on the floor to reduce the need for straining to reach
   c. in boxes where they will be out of the way
   d. all of the above
   e. none of the above

5. To clean a bathtub, you should
   a. bend over
   b. sit down on the floor
   c. kneel or use a low stool
   d. all of the above
   e. none of the above

4. Identify five common types of accidents in the home

In the following illustrations, circle everything you can find that is wrong in the picture.

32

Name: _____

5. List home fire safety guidelines and describe what to do in case of fire

Short Answer.

1. List four things that could be fire hazards.
   _____
   _____
   _____
   _____
   _____

2. What is important to remember about clothing while working near the stove?
   _____
   _____

3. How often should you check a smoke alarm? _____

4. RACE stands for:
   R: _____
   A: _____
   C: _____
   E: _____

5. PASS stands for:
   P: _____
   A: _____
   S: _____
   S: _____

6. List six guidelines for helping clients and family members exit a burning building safely.
   _____
   _____
   _____
   _____
   _____
   _____

6. Discuss the use of restraints and related problems

Short Answer.

1. When can restraints be used?
   _____
   _____
   _____
   _____
   _____

2. Look at the list of the negative effects of restraint use on page 80 in the textbook. Pick five of the negative effects and for each one you choose, describe why you think restraints could cause those problems.
   _____
   _____
   _____
   _____
   _____
   _____
   _____
   _____
   _____
   _____

7. Identify ways to reduce the risk of automobile accidents

Multiple Choice.

Circle the letter of the answer that best completes the statement.

1. When driving to a new client's house, you should:
   a. study the map while driving there
   b. plan your route before leaving
   c. look at a map only if you get lost
   d. all of the above
   e. none of the above

Name: _____

2. While driving, it is best to:
   a. keep your eyes on the road and your hands on the wheel
   b. listen to music to pass the time
   c. drive quickly so you will have more time at the client's home
   d. all of the above
   e. none of the above

3. When backing up in your car, you should:
   a. only use your rear view mirror
   b. back up quickly
   c. turn your head and look behind you
   d. all of the above
   e. none of the above

4. Driving at a safe speed means:
   a. obeying the speed limits
   b. making adjustments for road or weather conditions
   c. driving faster if it's snowing
   d. a and b only
   e. none of the above

5. Seat belts should always be worn because:
   a. they prevent accidents
   b. they help protect you in an accident
   c. they make you look professional
   d. all of the above
   e. none of the above

8. Identify guidelines for using your car on the job

True or False.

Mark each statement with either a "T" for true or an "F" for false.

1. _____ It is not necessary for you to keep track of the miles you drive for work.
2. _____ You should get your car serviced and check the tires regularly.
3. _____ Proof of registration should be kept in your car at all times.
4. _____ Keep proof of insurance at home where it will be safe.
5. _____ Put valuables under a seat or in the trunk if you must leave them in the car.
6. _____ Lock all your doors while driving and when leaving your car.

9. Identify guidelines for working in high-crime areas

Scenarios.

Circle the letter of the answer that best completes the question.

1. You are a home health aide going to visit a client who lives in a high-crime area. You have been to this client's apartment before, but today as you drive up you notice three strange men standing on the sidewalk in front of your client's apartment. They are watching you as you slow down in front of your client's apartment. What do you do?
   a. Ignore them and park your car.
   b. Keep driving past and find a phone to call your supervisor.
   c. Stop and ask them what they are doing in front of your client's apartment.
   d. none of the above

2. You are getting ready to leave a client's home as it begins to get dark. Your client lives in a large house on a street that is not well-lit. You have parked next to the nearest street light, which is two houses down.

   What should you do on your way to your car?
   a. Walk purposefully and confidently.
   b. Carry your keys in your hand.
   c. Hold your purse or bag close to your body.
   d. all of the above

7

Emergency Care and Disaster Preparation

1. Demonstrate how to recognize and respond to medical emergencies

Crossword.

Across

1. If the person is unable to respond, he may be _____.
5. If the injured person panics, _____ to him and tell him what actions are being taken to help him.
8. Make sure you are not in _____.
10. After an emergency, report the _____ only.

Down

2. When you come upon an emergency situation, remain calm, act quickly, and _____ clearly.
3. Notice the _____.
4. Once the emergency is over, you will have to file an _____ report.
6. Falls, _____, and cuts can be emergencies when they are severe.
7. When in doubt, call for _____.
9. Be _____ and confident to help reassure the injured person that he is being taken care of.

2. Demonstrate knowledge of first aid procedures

True or False.

Mark each statement with either a "T" for true or an "F" for false.

1. _____ CPR is an important skill for home health aides to learn.
2. _____ You should perform CPR on an unconscious victim even if you are not properly trained.
3. _____ You can contact the Red Cross to schedule a CPR training class.
4. _____ Performing CPR incorrectly cannot further injure a person.
5. _____ Rescue breathing can help in an emergency situation.
6. _____ Brain damage generally occurs 20 minutes after the heart stops beating and the lungs stop breathing.
7. _____ To give a chest compression, you must push in 1 1/2 to 2 inches with each compression.

Name: _____

8. _____ The Heimlich maneuver is a procedure used for choking.

Multiple Choice.

Circle the letter of the answer that best completes the statement or answers the question.

9. Signs of shock include:
   a. pale or bluish skin
   b. extreme thirst
   c. happiness
   d. none of the above
   e. a and c only

10. To control bleeding, you should:
    a. use your bare hands to stop it
    b. lower the wound below the heart
    c. hold a thick pad or clean cloth against the wound and press down hard
    d. none of the above
    e. all of the above

11. Which kind of burn involves just the outer layer of skin?
    a. first degree
    b. second degree
    c. third degree
    d. a and c
    e. all of the above

12. Which of the following are treatments for accidental poisoning?
    a. ipecac syrup
    b. activated charcoal
    c. Epsom salts
    d. all of the above
    e. none of the above

13. To treat a minor burn, you should:
    a. use ointment
    b. use grease, such as butter
    c. use ice water
    d. all of the above
    e. none of the above

14. Which of the following is true about assisting a person having a seizure?
    a. Give the person a glass of water to drink.
    b. Hold the person down if he or she is shaking severely.
    c. Move furniture away to prevent injury to the person.
    d. Open the person's mouth to move the tongue to the side.
    e. none of the above

15. If a person faints, you should:
    a. lower him to the floor
    b. position him on his side
    c. elevate his legs one inch
    d. help him stand up immediately
    e. none of the above

16. If a client falls, you should:
    a. wait until the end of the day to report the fall
    b. make client as comfortable as possible
    c. look for broken bones
    d. none of the above
    e. b and c

3. Identify emergency evacuation procedures

Short Answer.

List four ways to plan for an evacuation procedure.

_____
_____
_____
_____
_____
_____
_____
_____
_____
_____

4. Demonstrate knowledge of disaster procedures

Multiple Choice.

Circle the letter of the answer that best completes the statement.

1. A disaster kit should be assembled before disaster strikes. Disaster supplies include:
   a. an extra set of car keys and a change of clothing
   b. a television set
   c. cosmetics and a hair dryer
   d. three pair of shoes
   e. none of the above

2. In a disaster, stay informed by:
   a. running out to buy a newspaper
   b. going outside to find your neighbors
   c. listening to a radio
   d. calling your psychic
   e. none of the above

3. If a disaster is forecast, be prepared by:
   a. turning off your cell phone
   b. cleaning your house
   c. knowing how to start a fire
   d. wearing appropriate clothing and shoes
   e. none of the above

Name: _____   37

8

Physical, Psychological, and Social Health

1. Identify basic human needs

Short Answer.

1. Complete your own hierarchy of needs below. Some of the examples have already been completed for you.

   Maslow's Hierarchy of Needs

   Need
   a. Need for self-actualization
   b. Need for self-esteem
   c. Need for love
   d. Safety and security needs
   e. Physical needs

   Example
   a. I need the chance to learn new things.
   b. I need to know that I am doing a good job.
   c. _____
   d. _____
   e. _____

2. How do you think you would feel if you did not feel loved or understood?

   _____
   _____
   _____
   _____

2. Define holistic care

Short Answer.

In your own words, briefly define holistic care.

_____
_____
_____
_____
_____
_____

3. Identify ways to help clients meet their spiritual needs

Mark an "X" next to examples of good ways to assist clients with their spiritual needs.

1. _____ A client tells you that he cannot drink milk with his hamburger due to his religious beliefs. He asks you for some water instead. You take the milk away and bring him some water.

2. _____ A client tells you she is a Baptist and wants to know if you will call the local Baptist church to find out when the next service will be. "A Baptist?" you ask. "Why don't you just attend a Catholic service instead? I'm a Catholic and my church is close by."

3. _____ A client asks you to read a passage from his Bible. He tells you that it will comfort him. You open the Bible and begin to read.

4. _____ A client wants to see a rabbi. You call the rabbi he wants to see.

5. _____ You see a Buddha statue in a client's bedroom. You laugh and tell the client, "I couldn't keep this next to my bed. It would make me laugh too much."

6. _____ A spiritual leader is visiting with a client. You quietly leave the room and shut the door.

7. ____ A client tells you he is Muslim. You begin to explain Christianity to him and ask him to attend a Presbyterian service just to see what it's like.

8. ____ A client tells you that she doesn't believe in God. You do believe in God but do not argue with her. You listen quietly as she tells you her reasons.

4. Discuss family roles and their significance in health care

Short Answer.

1. List three types of families.

   _____

   _____

   _____

   _____

2. What kind of family did you grow up in?

   _____

   _____

   _____

   _____

   _____

   _____

5. Describe personal adjustments of the individual and family to illness and disability

Short Answer.

List three adjustments that family members may need to make due to the client's illness or disability.

_____

_____

_____

_____

6. Identify community resources for individual and family health

Short Answer.

1. If your client or the family asks you for more help, you should:

   _____

   _____

2. If you think your client or the family needs more help, but they do not ask, you should:

   _____

   _____

7. List ways to respond to emotional needs of clients and their families

Short Answer.

1. List three good ways to respond to clients or family members who come to you with problems or needs.

   _____

   _____

   _____

   _____

   _____

   _____

   _____

Multiple Choice.

Circle the letter of the answer that best completes the question.

2. You arrive at your client's house to find the wife, Mrs. McNabb, upset and close to tears. She tells you that her husband simply won't eat his breakfast. When you ask what she served him for breakfast, she begins to cry. What is the best thing to do?

   a. Tell her not to cry.

   b. Ask her why she is crying over something so unimportant.

   c. Reassure her that you are here to help.

Name: _____

3. You encourage Mrs. McNabb to talk to you about what is bothering her, and she confesses that she is feeling very overwhelmed. What is the best thing to say to her?
    a. "I know just how you feel. My kids are a handful, too."
    b. "It sounds like you are under a lot of stress. Can I help in some way?"
    c. "Well, I work two jobs myself, and it's no big deal."

4. Mrs. McNabb asks if you can stay longer during your visits to help her out with the cooking and cleaning. What is the best thing to say to her?
    a. I'll talk to my supervisor and see what she says. Maybe we can work something out.
    b. You should call a maid service to help you. Here's the phone book.
    c. I'm sorry, but I can't do that because it's not on the care plan.

9

The Human Body in Health and Disease

1. Describe the integumentary system

Fill in the Blank.

1. The largest organ and system in the body is the _____.

2. Skin prevents _____ to internal organs.

3. Skin also prevents the loss of too much _____, which is essential to life.

4. The skin is also a _____ that feels heat, cold, pain, touch, and pressure.

5. Blood vessels _____, or widen, when the outside temperature is too high.

6. Blood vessels _____, or close, when the outside temperature is too cold.

True or False.

Mark each statement with either a "T" for true or an "F" for false.

7. _____ Pressure sores cannot be prevented.

8. _____ Pressure sores usually occur in areas of the body where bone is close to the skin.

9. _____ The term "shearing" means lubricating dry skin.

10. _____ Another name for pressure sores is decubitus ulcers.

11. _____ Common sites for pressure sores are the chest, nose, and hands.

Labeling.

For each position shown list the areas at risk for pressure sores.

Prone Position

a.   b.   c.   d.   e.   f.

12. Prone Position
    a. _____
    b. _____
    c. _____
    d. _____
    e. _____
    f. _____

Supine Position

a.   b.   c.   d.   e.

13. Supine Position
    a. _____
    b. _____
    c. _____
    d. _____
    e. _____

Lateral Position

a.   b.   c.   d.   e.   f.   g.

14. Lateral Position
    a. _____
    b. _____
    c. _____
    d. _____
    e. _____
    f. _____
    g. _____

Name: _____

41

Short Answer.

15. List five signs and symptoms to observe and report about the integumentary system.

_____
_____
_____
_____
_____

2. Describe the musculoskeletal system

Short Answer.

1. What can range of motion exercises help prevent?

_____
_____
_____

2. List five of the signs to observe and report about the musculoskeletal system.

_____
_____
_____
_____
_____

Read each of the following. Decide if it is describing a fracture "F", osteoporosis "O", or arthritis "A".

3. _____ Signs and symptoms include low back pain and stooped posture.

4. _____ It occurs most commonly in women after menopause.

5. _____ It is a broken bone.

6. _____ It is the inflammation or swelling of a joint.

7. _____ To treat this, bones are held immobile (by a cast) until the bone can fuse itself back together.

8. _____ This disease causes bone to become porous and brittle.

9. _____ This disease can be prevented by adding extra calcium to the diet.

10. _____ The process of bones fusing back together takes longer with the elderly than with younger people.

3. Describe the nervous system

Crossword.

Across

3. The nervous system also _____ and interprets information from the environment outside the human body.

6. The peripheral nervous system deals with the outer part of the body, via the _____ that extend throughout the body.

Down

1. The nervous system is the _____ center and

2. _____ center of the body.

4. It controls and coordinates all body _____.

5. The central nervous system is composed of the _____ and spinal cord.

42

Name: _____

Matching.

For each of the following terms, write the letter of the correct definition from the list below.

1. _____ Alzheimer's disease
2. _____ Cerebral palsy
3. _____ CVA or stroke
4. _____ Dementia
5. _____ Epilepsy
6. _____ Multiple sclerosis
7. _____ Parkinson's disease
8. _____ Spinal cord injuries

a. This is an illness in which the myelin sheath that covers the nerves, spinal cord, and white matter of the brain breaks down over time.

b. This is a general term that refers to changes in the brain that alter personality and impair the ability to think and remember.

c. This illness causes a section of the brain to degenerate slowly and progressively.

d. This is a result of an injury to the cerebrum that occurs during pregnancy or the birth process.

e. This is an illness of the brain that produces seizures, which can range in severity from mild to violent.

f. This is an example of dementia with an unknown cause. It cannot be cured, is irreversible, and gets progressively worse.

g. The extent of these depends on the force of the impact and where on the spinal cord the injury is located.

h. This can cause sudden paresis (weakness) or paralysis (immobility) of certain parts of the body.

Short Answer.

9. List eight signs and symptoms to observe and report about the nervous system.

_____

_____
_____
_____
_____
_____
_____
_____
_____
_____

Fill in the Blank.

Fill in the blanks with the words listed below.

cataracts   otitis media
deafness   vertigo
glaucoma

10. _____ is the partial or complete loss of hearing. It can be the result of heredity, disease, or injury.

11. Milky or cloudy spots that develop in the eye and impair vision are _____. They can be surgically removed.

12. Dizziness which is usually the result of an inner ear disturbance or caused by diseases of the brain is _____.

13. _____ is an infection of the middle ear that can be caused by a variety of microorganisms.

14. The condition in which the fluid inside the eyeball is unable to drain, increasing pressure inside the eye and causing damage, is called _____.

Short Answer.

15. List two signs and symptoms to observe and report about the eyes and ears.

_____
_____
_____
_____
_____

Name: _____

43

4. Describe the circulatory or cardiovascular system

Multiple Choice.

Circle the letter of the answer that best completes the statement or answers the question.

1. The two upper chambers of the heart are called:
   a. veins
   b. cells
   c. left atrium and right atrium
   d. the pericardium
   e. none of the above

2. During the resting phase, or diastole, of the heart:
   a. ventricles pump blood through the blood vessels
   b. the heart begins beating rapidly until the next contraction
   c. circulation stops
   d. the chambers fill with blood
   e. none of the above

3. Which of the following is one of the functions that the circulatory system performs?
   a. senses and interprets information from the environment
   b. supplies food, oxygen, and hormones to cells
   c. removes waste products from cells
   d. both b and c
   e. none of the above

Crossword.

Across

5. Peripheral vascular disease is a disease in which the legs, feet, arms, or hands do not have enough blood _____.

Down

1. _____ is a hardening and narrowing of the blood vessels.

2. Hypertension is also known as _____.

3. Myocardial infarction is also known as a _____.

4. Congestive heart failure occurs when the heart is no longer able to _____ effectively.

6. _____ is a squeezing pain or feeling of pressure in the chest, left arm, or jaw.

5. Describe the respiratory system

Fill in the Blank.

1. Respiration is the body taking in _____ and removing _____.

2. It involves _____ and _____.

3. The _____ accomplish this process.

44

4. _____ is a chronic inflammatory disease. It occurs when the respiratory system is hyper-reactive to irritants, infection, cold air, or allergens such as pollen and dust.

5. _____ is an irritation and inflammation of the lining of the bronchi.

6. _____ is the development of abnormal cells or tumors in the lungs.

7. Symptoms of _____ include coughing, low-grade fever, shortness of breath, and bloody sputum.

8. For most people, _____ can be dealt with by the body's immune system and by rest, fluids, and antibiotics if the infection is bacterial.

9. Four chronic lung diseases are grouped under _____.

10. _____ can be caused by a bacterial, viral, or fungal infection. Acute inflammation occurs in a portion of lung tissue.

Short Answer.

11. List five signs and symptoms to observe and report about the respiratory system.

_____
_____
_____
_____
_____

6. Describe the urinary system

Short Answer.

1. How does urine pass out of the body?

_____
_____

2. What does urine do for the body?

_____
_____
_____
_____

True or False.

Mark each statement with either a "T" for true or an "F" for false.

3. _____ Cystitis is more common in men.

4. _____ Calculi, or kidney stones, form when urine crystallizes in the kidneys.

5. _____ Kidney dialysis is used for cleaning mucous from the lungs.

6. _____ When someone has a UTI they may experience a painful burning sensation during urination and the frequent feeling of needing to urinate.

7. _____ To avoid infection, women should wipe the perineal area from back to front after elimination.

8. _____ Kidney stones can be the result of a vitamin deficiency or mineral imbalance.

9. _____ Nephritis may cause rusty-colored urine and a decrease in urine output.

10. _____ Excessive salt in the diet can cause damage to the kidneys.

Short Answer.

11. List five signs and symptoms to observe and report about the urinary system.

_____
_____
_____
_____
_____
_____

Name: _____

7. Describe the gastrointestinal or digestive system

Crossword.

Across

2. To prevent heartburn and gastric reflux, provide an extra pillow to make the client's body more _____ during sleep.

5. Gastric reflux occurs when stomach contents pass through the _____ into the lungs.

6. Ulcerative colitis is a chronic inflammatory disease of the large _____ that usually occurs in young adults.

8. Raw sores in the stomach or small intestine are called _____.

12. A diet of bananas, rice, apples, and tea/toast is called the _____ diet.

13. Constipation occurs when the feces move too slowly through the intestine as the result of decreased _____ intake and poor diet.

15. Good _____ is important in the treatment of hepatitis.

16. Cancer of the gastrointestinal tract is _____ cancer.

Down

1. Heartburn is a result of a weakening of the _____ muscle.

3. Hepatitis B and C can lead to _____ and liver cancer.

4. A condition where the skin and body fluids appear yellow is _____.

7. _____ are enlarged veins in the rectum that cause itching and burning.

9. If heartburn occurs frequently and remains untreated, it can cause scarring or _____.

10. Treatment of _____ often includes increasing the amount of fiber eaten.

11. Clients with peptic ulcers should avoid _____.

14. _____ is the frequent elimination of liquid or semi-liquid feces.

16. Surgical treatment of ulcerative colitis may include a _____.

Short Answer.

17. List nine signs and symptoms to observe and report about the gastrointestinal system.

_____
_____
_____
_____
_____
_____
_____
_____
_____

8. Describe the endocrine system

Fill in the Blank.

1. Signs and symptoms of diabetes include increased _____ and _____ production.

2. _____ occurs when the thyroid produces too little thyroid hormone and the body processes slow down.

3. Diabetes is a chronic disease that has two forms: _____ and _____.

4. Weight loss, nervousness, and hyperactivity occur with _____.

5. When sugar builds up in the blood and cannot get to the cells, it makes it difficult for the body to process carbohydrates, _____, and proteins.

Short Answer.

6. List eight signs and symptoms to observe and report about the endocrine system immediately.

_____
_____
_____
_____
_____
_____
_____
_____

9. Describe the reproductive system

True or False.

Mark each statement with either a "T" for true or an "F" for false.

1. _____ Gonorrhea can be treated with antibiotics and is easier to detect in men than in women.

2. _____ People with herpes always experience repeated outbreaks.

3. _____ Condoms can reduce the chances of being infected or passing on some STDs.

4. _____ Gonorrhea can cause sterility in both men and women.

5. _____ Symptoms of chlamydia include yellow or white discharge from the penis or vagina and a burning sensation during urination.

6. _____ Chlamydia cannot be treated with antibiotics.

7. _____ If left untreated, syphilis can cause brain damage or death.

8. _____ Most women infected with gonorrhea show many early symptoms.

9. _____ Benign prostatic hypertrophy is a fairly common disorder that occurs in both women and men as they age.

10. _____ STDs can only be transmitted by sexual intercourse.

11. _____ Herpes is caused by a virus and cannot be treated with antibiotics.

12. _____ Chancres, or open sores, that develop on the penis make it easier for syphilis to be detected in men than in women.

13. _____ Penicillin can be used to treat syphilis.

Short Answer.

14. List seven signs and symptoms to observe and report about the reproductive system.

_____
_____
_____
_____
_____
_____
_____

10. Describe the immune and lymphatic systems

Short Answer.

1. What two systems are related to the lymphatic system?

_____
_____

2. What is lymph?

_____
_____
_____

3. What is the difference between nonspecific immunity and specific immunity?

_____
_____
_____
_____
_____

4. List three signs and symptoms to observe and report about the immune system.

_____
_____
_____
_____

10

Human Development and Aging

1. Describe the stages of human development and identify common disorders for each group

Infancy, Birth to Twelve Months

True or False.

Mark each statement with either a "T" for true or an "F" for false.

1. _____ An infant takes three years to be able to move around, communicate basic needs, and feed himself.

2. _____ Infants develop from the hands to the head.

3. _____ Caregivers should encourage infants to stand as soon as they can hold their heads up.

4. _____ Studies show that putting an infant to sleep on its back can reduce the risk of sudden infant death syndrome (SIDS).

Short Answer.

5. List three common disorders of infancy.

_____

_____

_____

_____

Childhood

True or False.

Mark each statement with either a "T" for true or an "F" for false.

1. _____ Tantrums are common among toddlers.

2. _____ The best way to deal with tantrums is to give the toddler what he wants.

3. _____ Pre-schoolaged children are too young to know right from wrong.

4. _____ Children aged three to six are beginning to learn how to play cooperatively with each other.

5. _____ From the ages of six to eight years, most children begin to go through puberty.

6. _____ School-age children develop cognitively and socially.

Short Answer.

7. List three common disorders of childhood.

_____

_____

_____

_____

Adolescence

True or False.

Mark each statement with either a "T" for true or an "F" for false.

1. _____ Puberty is the stage of growth when secondary sex characteristics, such as body hair, appear.

2. _____ Most adolescents do not struggle with peer acceptance or self-image or self-esteem.

3. _____ Adolescents may be moody due to changing hormones and peer pressure.

4. _____ Eating disorders cannot be life-threatening.

5. _____ Due to changes they are experiencing, adolescents may become depressed and may attempt suicide.

Name: _____

Short Answer.

6. List three common disorders of adolescence.

_____
_____
_____

Adulthood

True or False.

Mark each statement with either a "T" for true or an "F" for false.

1. _____ By eighteen years of age, most young adults have stopped developing physically, psychologically, and socially.

2. _____ One developmental task that most young adults undertake is to choose an occupation or career.

3. _____ A "mid-life crisis" is a period of unrest when a person has an unconscious desire for change and fulfillment of unmet goals.

4. _____ Middle adults usually do not experience any physical changes due to aging.

5. _____ Menopause is a condition in middle adult women that occurs when the ovaries begin to secrete hormones.

6. _____ By the time a person reaches late adulthood, his or her body has stopped changing due to the effects of aging.

2. Distinguish between fact (what is true) and fallacy (what is not true) about the aging process

True or False.

Mark each statement with either a "T" for true or an "F" for false.

1. _____ Older adults have different capabilities depending upon their health.

2. _____ As people age, they often become lonely, forgetful, and slow.

3. _____ Diseases and illness are not a normal part of aging.

4. _____ Many older adults can lead active and healthy lives.

3. Discuss normal changes of aging and list care guidelines

Multiple Choice.

Circle the letter of the answer that best completes the statement or answers the question.

1. Older adults experience changes in their skin due to aging because:
   a. much of the fatty layer beneath the skin is lost
   b. they develop allergies to skin care products
   c. circulation to the skin is reduced
   d. both a and c
   e. none of the above

2. Changes to the musculoskeletal system include:
   a. brittle bones
   b. stiff joints
   c. weaker muscles
   d. all of the above
   e. none of the above

3. For clients with poor vision, you should:
   a. discourage wearing sunglasses outside
   b. keep eyeglasses clean
   c. provide good lighting
   d. both a and c
   e. both b and c

4. For clients who are hard of hearing, you should:
   a. speak in a low-pitched voice
   b. exaggerate your movements as you speak
   c. shout to be heard
   d. all of the above
   e. none of the above

5. For clients with a poor sense of taste and smell, you should:
   a. make sure food in the house is fresh
   b. make sure there are working smoke and carbon monoxide detectors in the home
   c. only feed them spicy foods
   d. all of the above
   e. a and b

6. Which of the following is true about clients who have a poor sense of touch?
   a. Poor sense of touch may be caused by decreased circulation and dry skin.
   b. A client who is confined to bed is at risk for developing pressure sores.
   c. Clients cannot tell if something is too hot. You must be careful with hot drinks and hot water.
   d. all of the above

7. Clients with heart conditions should:
   a. exercise vigorously to regain strength
   b. avoid vigorous activity
   c. climb stairs as much as possible
   d. all of the above
   e. none of the above

8. If your client is cold due to poor circulation, the best thing she can do is:
   a. use a hot water bottle or heating pad
   b. go without slippers
   c. wear layers of clothing and turn the thermostat up
   d. all of the above
   e. none of the above

9. Shortness of breath due to normal aging changes is caused by:
   a. exercising too hard
   b. cancer of the lungs
   c. fewer alveoli for oxygen/carbon dioxide exchange
   d. all of the above
   e. none of the above

10. Older clients may need to urinate more frequently due to
    a. the bladder not being able to hold as much urine
    b. drinking more fluids than younger adults
    c. incontinence
    d. all of the above
    e. none of the above

11. Incontinence:
    a. is a normal part of aging
    b. could be a sign of illness
    c. occurs when a person drinks too much fluid
    d. all of the above
    e. none of the above

12. Constipation could be the result of:
    a. slower digestion process due to aging
    b. eating too much food during the day
    c. not getting enough water or fiber
    d. all of the above
    e. both a and c

13. Because the pancreas function lessens due to aging, some clients may:
    a. develop diabetes
    b. need to take insulin to regulate blood sugar
    c. have special instructions in the care plan
    d. all of the above
    e. none of the above

14. Normal changes in the reproductive system due to aging often result in:
    a. loss of sexual drive
    b. decrease of mucous secretions in the vagina for women
    c. inappropriate sexual advances
    d. all of the above
    e. none of the above

15. Which of the following is a result of a weakened immune system due to normal changes of aging?
    a. may take longer to recover from an illness
    b. developing HIV
    c. developing anemia
    d. all of the above
    e. none of the above

16. Which of the following is a result of decreased number and size of lymph nodes due to normal changes of aging?
    a. fewer infections
    b. less able to contract a fever
    c. developing diabetes
    d. all of the above
    e. none of the above

17. Insomnia, withdrawal, and moodiness could all be signs of:
    a. anorexia
    b. depression
    c. confusion
    d. all of the above
    e. none of the above

18. One way you can help your clients adjust to lifestyle changes due to aging is to:
    a. listen to them
    b. ensure that their home is safe
    c. care about their feelings
    d. all of the above
    e. none of the above

19. What is the most important thing to do if you observe any changes in your client's condition?
    a. report it to your supervisor
    b. report it to your supervisor
    c. report it to your supervisor
    d. report it to your supervisor
    e. all of the above

4. Identify attitudes and living habits that promote good health

Short Answer.

List six things you can do to encourage your clients to stay active, maintain self-esteem, and live independently.

_____

_____

_____

_____

_____

_____

_____

_____

_____

_____

5. List ways to recognize and report elder abuse and neglect

Short Answer.

1. What are some possible reasons why elderly people may be abused?

_____

_____

_____

_____

_____

2. What must a home health aide do if he or she suspects or witnesses elder abuse?

_____

_____

_____

_____

_____

_____

6. Identify community resources available to help the elderly

Project.

Find information about three agencies or organizations in your area serving the needs of the elderly. List their names and what services they offer below.

_____
_____
_____
_____
_____
_____
_____
_____
_____
_____

Name: _____

11

Dying, Death and Hospice

1. Discuss the stages of dying

Multiple Choice.

Circle the letter of the answer that best completes the statement or answers the question.

1. Mrs. Levine, a resident, prays about her terminal illness. She promises God that she will make peace with her sister, whom she has not seen in 20 years, if she is allowed to live. Which stage of dying is Mrs. Levine going through?
   a. denial
   b. anger
   c. bargaining
   d. depression
   e. acceptance

2. A terminally ill resident, Mr. Lucero, begins to yell at Peter, his nursing assistant. He says that Peter never took good care of him. He blames Peter for a lack of proper care. Peter does not take it personally because he realizes that Mr. Lucero may be going through the _____ stage of dying.
   a. denial
   b. anger
   c. bargaining
   d. depression
   e. acceptance

3. Resident Amy Scott is dying. Her priest visits her at her request. When he asks her if there is anything he can do to help her get things in order, she tells him she has no idea what he is talking about. Instead she begins to tell him the latest news about her son. Mrs. Scott is experiencing:
   a. denial
   b. anger
   c. bargaining
   d. depression
   e. acceptance

4. A terminally ill resident, John Castillo, visits with his family. He discusses his funeral arrangements with them. He lets them know that he is concerned about their well-being after he is gone. He says he wants to spend as much time as possible with them before he dies. Mr. Castillo is going through the _____ stage of dying.
   a. denial
   b. anger
   c. bargaining
   d. depression
   e. acceptance

5. A terminally ill resident cries constantly. She doesn't want to talk to anyone. She may be experiencing the _____ stage of dying.
   a. denial
   b. anger
   c. bargaining
   d. depression
   e. acceptance

2. Describe the grief process

Word Search.

Complete each of the following sentences and find your answers in the word search.

1. Even if a death is expected, family members and friends may still experience _____.

2. When a person dies, family members or friends may cope initially by refusing to

believe that they are grieving. This is referred to as _____.

3. Often people experience _____ about what they did or did not do for the dying person. They may wish they had done more for the dying person.

4. Experiencing _____ towards God, doctors, or even towards the person who died is a normal part of the grief process.

5. Sometimes family members and/or friends may _____ things they said or did not say to a person who has died.

6. Experiencing _____ or depression is very common after a person dies. Missing someone who has died or having a sense of _____ is also a normal part of the grief process.

l	y	g	d	k	o	t	s	l	g	d	z	n	t
o	o	t	p	k	w	e	a	d	a	r	o	l	j
s	w	n	q	o	e	r	d	u	w	i	i	e	u
k	l	z	e	y	i	g	n	o	a	u	n	x	n
b	q	c	x	l	e	e	e	v	g	g	s	e	g
j	m	w	o	l	i	r	s	u	s	e	j	t	d
p	r	l	y	c	f	n	s	w	y	s	v	a	w
e	a	w	c	i	c	f	e	n	t	g	u	k	e
p	a	y	y	o	u	w	s	s	k	c	o	h	s
r	c	e	k	c	r	w	e	u	s	t	m	q	q
d	y	w	l	e	e	s	w	o	w	y	e	z	u
p	z	d	v	z	g	d	v	c	b	v	r	a	b
s	o	a	j	d	n	m	x	b	e	i	t	n	y
u	j	x	h	j	a	b	w	r	s	r	k	j	f

3. Discuss how feelings and attitudes about death differ

Short Answer.

1. Have you ever experienced the death of a loved one? If so, what are some of the emotions you felt?

_____

_____

Name: _____

_____
_____
_____
_____
_____
_____

2. What, if any, religious beliefs do you subscribe to? How do they influence your feelings about death?

_____
_____
_____
_____
_____
_____
_____
_____

3. What cultural background do you have? What cultures are you familiar with? Briefly describe how your culture or other cultures feel about death.

_____
_____
_____
_____
_____
_____
_____
_____
_____
_____

4. Explain common signs of approaching death

Mark an "X" next to the signs of approaching death

1. _____ abundance of physical activity

2. _____ body temperature that is above or below normal

3. _____ cold, pale skin

Name: _____   55

4. _____ disorientation
5. _____ healthy skin tone
6. _____ heightened sense of touch
7. _____ impaired speech
8. _____ incontinence
9. _____ perspiration
10. _____ strong pulse

5. Discuss how to care for a dying client

Crossword.

Across

1. _____ care means care of the body after death.
3. _____ perspiring clients often.
6. Clients may not be able to communicate that they are in _____. Observe your clients for signs and report them.
7. Changes of position, back massage, _____ care,
8. _____ care, and proper body alignment may help to relieve pain.
10. _____ may be one of the most important things you can do for a client who is dying.

Down

2. After death, do not remove any _____ or other equipment.
4. _____ is usually the last sense to leave the body.
5. Observe _____ to anticipate a client's needs.
9. After a person dies, drainage pads are needed most often under the head and/or under the _____.
11. Keep the room _____ lighted and without glare.

6. Define the goals of a hospice program

True or False.

Mark each statement with either a "T" for true or an "F" for false.

1. _____ Hospice care can be provided in a hospital or in the home.
2. _____ Caregivers should insist that family members take breaks.
3. _____ Often, clients who are dying do not care about independence anymore.
4. _____ The goals of hospice care are the comfort and dignity of the client.
5. _____ It is important in hospice care to make clients comfortable, rather than keeping an eye to recovery.

Short Answer.

6. Look at the Dying Person's Bill of Rights on page 135 of your textbook. Pick three rights that you feel would be most important to you personally. Briefly describe why they would be important to you.

_____

_____

4. The services provided by volunteers include caring for the home or family of a dying person, driving or doing errands, and _____.

9. Discuss the importance of caring for yourself when working in hospice care

Short Answer.

1. How do you alleviate stress in your life?

2. What sorts of things do you do to take care of yourself?

7. Identify special skills and attitudes helpful in hospice work

Short Answer.

List five helpful attitudes for hospice work.

8. Describe the role of the hospice volunteer

Fill in the Blank.

1. According to the National Hospice and Palliative Care Organization, there are now more than _____ hospices across the country.

2. Hospice volunteers go through a _____ program to prepare them for hospice work.

3. Volunteers give more than _____ hours of their time each year to help.

12

Transfers, Ambulation, and Positioning

1. **Explain the guidelines for safely transferring and positioning clients**

   Multiple Choice.

   Circle the letter of the answer that best completes the statement or answers the question.

   1. Before a client who has been lying down moves to a standing position, he should:
      a. do a few sit-ups in bed to get used to the upright position
      b. sit up with his feet over the side of the bed for a moment, or dangle
      c. drink some water or other fluid
      d. all of the above
      e. none of the above

   2. If a client starts to fall, the best thing to do is:
      a. widen your stance and bring the client's body close to you
      b. catch the client under the arms to stop the fall
      c. allow the client to fall since you could be injured trying to break the fall
      d. all of the above
      e. none of the above

   3. If a client falls, what is the first thing you should do?
      a. help the client get up and into bed
      b. report it to your supervisor
      c. call for help if a family member is around
      d. all of the above
      e. none of the above

   4. A client who has some difficulty with balance but can bear weight on both legs should use a:
      a. walker
      b. cane
      c. wheelchair
      d. all of the above
      e. none of the above

   5. Your role in wheelchair transfers is to:
      a. make sure the client is safe and comfortable
      b. ask the client how you can assist
      c. check the client's alignment in the chair when the transfer is complete
      d. all of the above
      e. none of the above

2. **Explain the guidelines for safely positioning a client in each of the five basic positions**

   Labeling.

   Label each position below and describe comfort measures appropriate for each.

   1. _____

   Comfort measures: _____
   _____
   _____

2. _____

Comfort measures: _____
_____
_____
_____

3. _____

Comfort measures: _____
_____
_____
_____

4. _____

Comfort measures: _____
_____
_____
_____

5. _____

Comfort measures: _____
_____
_____
_____

Name: _____

Short Answer.

6. What is shearing?
_____
_____

7. What is logrolling?
_____
_____

3. List things you can do to help make your client comfortable

Labeling.

Label each positioning device and explain its purpose.

1. _____
_____
_____
_____

2. _____
_____
_____
_____

Name: _____

59

3. _____
_____
_____
_____

True or False.

Mark each statement with either a "T" for true or an "F" for false.

4. _____ In the past, physical restraints were intended to keep clients from wandering, becoming violent, or hurting themselves.

5. _____ You are allowed to use physical restraints on a client if he or she has been rude to you.

6. _____ If your client is in a physical restraint, you must check on him or her at least every half hour.

7. _____ A doctor must prescribe a restraint.

13

Personal Care Skills

1. Describe the home health aide's role in assisting clients with personal care

Short Answer.

1. List three things to observe when providing or assisting with personal care.

   _____

   _____

   _____

   _____

2. List three things to observe about a client's room after finishing a procedure.

   _____

   _____

   _____

   _____

2. Explain guidelines for assisting with bathing

Fill in the Blank.

1. A sturdy, water-resistant chair designed to be placed in the bathtub is called a _____ or _____ chair.

2. _____ promotes good health and well-being by removing the perspiration, dirt, oil, and dead skin cells that accumulate on the skin.

3. Before bathing any client or assisting with bathing, make sure the room is _____ enough.

4. The face, hands, _____, and perineum should be washed every day, but complete baths or showers can be taken every other day.

5. A transfer belt, tub chair, and safety bars are all examples of _____ which can make bathing easier and safer.

6. Some agencies only require HHAs to wear gloves during bathing for _____ care or if broken skin is present.

7. _____ or _____ bars are often installed to allow clients something to help them change position.

8. Older skin produces less _____ and oil.

9. Never leave an elderly person or young child _____ while in the bathtub.

10. The bed bath is an excellent time for _____ arms and legs and increasing _____.

3. Describe guidelines for assisting with grooming

True or False.

Mark each statement with either a "T" for true or an "F" for false.

1. _____ If a client wears regular clothes rather than nightclothes during the day, he or she is more likely to be sleepy.

2. _____ Clients should not choose their clothing for the day; you should pick it for them.

Name: _____

3. _____ Front-fastening bras are easier for clients to manage by themselves.

4. _____ When dressing a client who has a weakness or paralysis on one side, dress the stronger side first.

5. _____ Clients are never embarrassed to have people help them with grooming tasks.

6. _____ You should protect a client's privacy by never exposing more than you need to.

7. _____ If a client has a weaker left arm due to a stroke, refer to it as the "bad" arm.

4. Identify guidelines for good oral care

Short Answer.

1. How often should oral care be performed? When should it be done?

   _____
   _____
   _____
   _____

2. List six signs to observe and report about the mouth when performing oral care.

   _____
   _____
   _____
   _____
   _____
   _____

3. What is aspiration?

   _____
   _____
   _____
   _____

5. Explain care guidelines for hearing aids and prosthetic devices

True or False.

Mark each statement with either a "T" for true or an "F" for false.

1. _____ You must submerge a hearing aid in water in order to clean it.

2. _____ Clients should keep an extra battery for their hearing aid on hand.

3. _____ Wearing gloves is unnecessary when caring for an artificial eye.

4. _____ Prostheses are expensive, fitted pieces of equipment.

5. _____ Artificial eyes are held in by a special type of glue.

6. _____ When cleaning a hearing aid, you can generally use a little soap and water on a cloth.

7. _____ A prosthesis is a device that helps a client hear better.

8. _____ After rinsing the artificial eye, it should be placed far under the upper eyelid.

6. Explain guidelines for assisting with toileting

Labeling.

Label each assistive device below and explain its purpose.

1. _____

Purpose: _____

62

Name: _____

_____
_____
_____

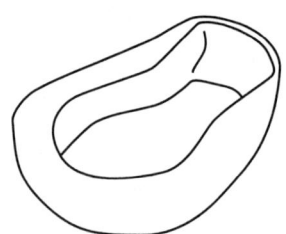

2. _____

Purpose: _____
_____
_____

3. _____

Purpose: _____
_____
_____
_____

4. _____

Purpose: _____
_____
_____
_____

7. Describe how to dispose of body wastes

Short Answer.

1. How must washcloths used to clean perineal areas be washed?

_____
_____
_____
_____

2. Why must you wear gloves when handling bedpans, urinals, or basins that contain wastes, including dirty bath water?

_____
_____
_____
_____
_____
_____
_____
_____

14

Core Healthcare Skills

1. Explain the importance of monitoring vital signs

Short Answer.

1. What can changes in vital signs indicate? Which changes should be immediately reported to a supervisor?

_____
_____
_____
_____
_____
_____
_____
_____

Labeling.

For each of the mercury-free thermometers shown below, write the temperature reading to the nearest tenth degree.

2. _____

3. _____

4. _____

5. _____

Multiple Choice.

Circle the letter of the answer that best answers the question.

6. Which of the following is the normal temperature range for the oral method?
   a. 96.6 - 98.6 degrees F
   b. 93.6 - 97.9 degrees F
   c. 98.6 - 100.6 degrees F
   d. 97.6 - 99.6 degrees F
   e. none of the above

7. Which of the following blood pressures falls within the normal range?
   a. 119/75
   b. 135/90
   c. 91/70
   d. 140/80
   e. all of the above

8. Which of the following thermometers is used to take a temperature from the ear?
   a. oral thermometer
   b. rectal thermometer
   c. axillary thermometer
   d. tympanic thermometer
   e. none of the above

9. Which of the following thermometers is used to take a temperature from the armpit?
   a. oral thermometer
   b. rectal thermometer
   c. axillary thermometer
   d. tympanic thermometer
   e. none of the above

10. Which temperature is considered to be the most accurate?
    a. oral
    b. rectal
    c. axillary
    d. tympanic
    e. none of the above

11. Under what condition should you not take an oral temperature on a person?
    a. if the person is unconscious
    b. if the person is confused or disoriented
    c. if the person is paralyzed from stroke
    d. all of the above
    e. none of the above

12. Why are mercury-free thermometers considered safer than the mercury thermometers?
    a. They do not contain mercury, which is a dangerous and toxic substance.
    b. They are smaller than mercury thermometers.
    c. They are read differently than mercury thermometers.
    d. all of the above
    e. none of the above

Short Answer.

13. What is the most common site for monitoring the pulse?

    _____

    _____

True or False.

Mark each statement with either a "T" for true or an "F" for false.

14. _____ An unusually high or low pulse rate does not necessarily indicate disease.

15. _____ A rapid pulse may result from dehydration or shock.

16. _____ It is best to measure the apical pulse on infants and small children because their pulse points are harder to find.

17. _____ The apical pulse is heard by listening directly over the wrist.

Fill in the Blank.

18. Breathing air into the lungs is also called _____.

19. Exhaling air out of the lungs is also called _____.

20. The normal respiration rate for adults ranges from _____ to _____ breaths per minute.

21. The normal respiration rate for infants ranges from _____ to _____ breaths per minute.

Short Answer.

22. Why is it important to observe your client's respirations without letting him or her know that is what you are doing?

    _____

    _____

    _____

Matching.

For each of the following terms, write the letter of the correct definition from the list.

23. _____ 100–139 mmHg
24. _____ 60–89 mmHg
25. _____ diastolic phase
26. _____ hypertension
27. _____ hypotension
28. _____ mmHg
29. _____ sphygmomanometer
30. _____ systolic phase

a. Blood pressure in the arteries when the heart is contracting
b. Low blood pressure

Name: _____

c. Blood pressure in the arteries when the heart is relaxed

d. High blood pressure

e. Blood pressure cuff

f. Normal range for diastolic blood pressure

g. Measuring unit used for blood pressure

h. Normal range for systolic blood pressure

Short Answer.

31. What questions should you ask to get the most accurate information if a client complains of pain?

_____
_____
_____
_____
_____
_____

32. List five measures to reduce a client's pain.

_____
_____
_____
_____
_____

2. List three types of specimens you may collect from a client

Short Answer.

1. List the three types of specimens you may have to collect from a client:

_____
_____
_____

2. Which type of specimen may require a 24-hour collection?

_____
_____
_____
_____

3. What is a "hat"?

_____
_____
_____

4. What is another term for "calculi"?

_____
_____
_____

3. Describe the importance of fluid balance and explain intake and output (I&O)

Short Answer.

1. A healthy person generally needs to take in about 64 to 96 oz. of fluid each day. How many cc is this? _____ to _____ cc. How many cups is this? _____ to _____ cups.

2. Mrs. Wyant drinks half of a glass of orange juice. You know that the glass holds about 1 cup of liquid. How many cc of orange juice did Mrs. Wyant drink?
_____

3. Mr. Bernicke just ate some chocolate pudding from a 6 oz. container. You measure the leftover pudding, which is about 35 cc. How many cc of pudding did Mr. Bernicke eat? _____

4. Miss Cahill has a bowl of soup for lunch. The soup bowl holds about 1 ½ cups of liquid. Convert this to cc. _____. Miss Cahill finishes most of her soup, but there is about 25 cc left. How many cc of soup did Miss Cahill eat? _____

66

5. List three guidelines to follow when a client vomits.

___

4. List six things to report to the supervisor about a client's catheter.

___

4. Describe the guidelines for catheter care

Short Answer.

1. Briefly define an indwelling catheter.

___

2. Briefly define an external or condom catheter.

___

3. List three guidelines to follow when working around clients with catheters.

___

5. Explain the benefits of warm and cold applications

Crossword.

Across

4. If you observe excessive, _____ pain,

6. _____, or numbness with warm or cold applications, report it to your supervisor.

Down

1. Heat relieves _____ and muscular tension. It reduces swelling, elevates the temperature in the tissues, and increases

2. _____.

3. bring down high _____.

Name: _____

5. Another type of heat application is a warm soak of the perineal area, which is also called a _____.

6. Cold applications can help stop _____.
They reduce swelling and pain, and

6. Explain how to apply non-sterile dressings

Short Answer.

What is the difference between sterile and non-sterile dressings?

_____
_____
_____
_____
_____
_____
_____
_____

7. Describe the purpose of anti-embolic hose

Short Answer.

What is the purpose of elastic stockings?

_____
_____
_____
_____
_____
_____
_____
_____
_____

8. Define the term ostomy and list care guidelines

True or False.

Mark each statement with either a "T" for true or an "F" for false.

1. _____ An ostomy is the surgical removal of part of the stomach.

2. _____ A stoma is an artificial opening in the abdomen through which stool is eliminated.

3. _____ In a colostomy, the stool will generally be semi-solid.

4. _____ In an ileostomy, the stool will generally be solid.

5. _____ The ostomy bag should be emptied and cleaned once a day.

Short Answer.

6. Why do you think a client with an ostomy might feel embarrassed about it?

_____
_____
_____
_____
_____
_____
_____
_____

15

Rehabilitation and Restorative Care

1. List goals of restorative home care

Short Answer.

List four goals of a restorative home care program.

_____
_____
_____
_____

2. Explain the home care rehabilitation model

Short Answer.

List five members of the team who may participate in a client's restorative care.

_____
_____
_____
_____
_____

3. Describe guidelines for assisting with restorative care

True or False.

Mark each statement with either a "T" for true or an "F" for false.

1. _____ You should downplay any setbacks a client experiences so he or she does not become discouraged.

2. _____ Your reactions and attitudes really do not affect a client's progress.

3. _____ If you can do a task faster than your client, you should do it yourself.

4. _____ Do not report any decline in a client's ability.

5. _____ Family members and clients will take cues from you on how to behave.

6. _____ Tasks are less overwhelming when they are broken down into small steps.

7. _____ It is important to report any signs of depression or mood changes in a client.

4. Describe how to assist with range of motion exercises

Matching.

For each of the following terms, write the letter of the correct definition from the list below.

1. _____ active assisted range of motion
2. _____ active range of motion
3. _____ contracture
4. _____ passive range of motion
5. _____ range of motion

a. The permanent and often painful stiffening of a joint and muscle, caused by immobility

b. Exercises performed by the client with some assistance and support

c. Exercises used by clients who are not able to move on their own

d. Exercises that put a particular joint through its full arc of motion

e. Exercises performed by the client himself, using his own muscle power

Name: _____

Labeling.

For each of the following illustrations, put the correct term of the exercise.

6. _____
_____
_____

7. _____
_____
_____

8. _____
_____
_____

9. _____
_____
_____

10. _____
_____
_____

11. _____
_____
_____

12. _____
_____
_____

13. _____
_____
_____

5. Explain guidelines for maintaining proper body alignment

Fill in the Blank.

1. Observe principles of _____. Remember that proper alignment is based on a straight _____. _____ or rolled or folded _____ may be needed to support the small of the back and raise the knees or head in the supine position.

2. Keep body parts in natural _____. In a natural hand position, the fingers are slightly _____. Use _____ to keep covers from resting on feet in the supine position.

3. Prevent external rotation of _____. Change _____ frequently to prevent muscle stiffness and pressure ulcers. Every _____ hours is usually adequate.

6. List important observations to make about changes in a client's skin

Short Answer.

List eight important observations to make about changes in a client's skin.

_____
_____
_____
_____
_____
_____
_____
_____
_____
_____
_____
_____

70

7. List guidelines for providing basic skin care and preventing pressure sores

Crossword.

Across

4. Reposition immobile clients at least every _____ hours.

3. Provide regular care for skin to keep it _____ and

6. _____.

5. A _____, chamois skin, or bed pad, absorbs moisture under the back and buttocks.

7. Avoid pulling the client across sheets during transfers or repositioning because it causes _____.

Down

1. _____ the skin frequently, using light, circular strokes to increase circulation.

4. Keep the bottom sheet _____ and free from wrinkles and the bed free

2. from _____.

5. Report changes you observe in a client's _____.

8. Describe the guidelines for caring for clients who have fractures or casts

Multiple Choice.

Circle the letter of the answer that best completes the statement.

1. When caring for a client who has a cast, _____ the extremity that is in a cast to help stop swelling.
   a. lower
   b. double bandage
   c. elevate
   d. shake
   e. none of the above

2. Keep the cast _____ at all times.
   a. dry
   b. wet
   c. hot
   d. pointed
   e. none of the above

3. Osteoporosis occurs more frequently in _____ people.
   a. young
   b. active
   c. elderly
   d. imprisoned
   e. none of the above

4. A wet cast is grey, dull, cool, and smells:
   a. fruity
   b. musty
   c. spicy
   d. chocolatey
   e. none of the above

5. A bone must be _____ to allow the fusion of fractured parts.
   a. lowered
   b. surgically repaired
   c. wet
   d. immobilized
   e. none of the above

6. Signs and symptoms of a fracture include:
   a. heat
   b. cold
   c. swelling
   d. dryness
   e. none of the above

Name: _____ 71

7. Fractures are broken bones caused by:
   a. accidents
   b. talking
   c. osteoporosis
   d. both a and c
   e. none of the above

8. You can place a wet cast on _____ so that its shape is not altered as it dries.
   a. a metal surface
   b. pillows
   c. concrete
   d. a wood floor
   e. none of the above

9. List the guidelines for caring for a client who has a hip fracture

True or False.

Mark each statement with either a "T" for true or an "F" for false.

1. _____ Most fractured hips require surgery.
2. _____ You should provide ROM exercises for a leg on the side of a hip replacement when you feel it is necessary.
3. _____ A hip fracture is not really a serious injury.
4. _____ Elderly people heal slowly.
5. _____ Home health aides may disconnect traction assembly.
6. _____ A client recovering from a hip replacement should not sit with his or her legs crossed. The hip cannot be at less than a 90-degree angle.
7. _____ Dress a client recovering from a hip replacement starting with the unaffected side first.
8. _____ A red or warm incision after hip replacement surgery must be reported to the supervisor.

10. List ways to adapt the environment for people with physical limitations

Short Answer.

Choose an adaptive device from Figure 15-33 in the textbook that you did not choose for the Chapter Review. Describe how it might help a client who is recovering from or adapting to a physical condition.

_____
_____
_____
_____
_____
_____
_____

11. Identify reasons clients lose bowel or bladder control

Word Search.

Complete each of the following sentences and find your answers in the word search.

e	k	i	a	t	f	u	u	y	e	x	n	r	n
z	g	i	p	e	t	b	s	j	r	c	a	j	x
l	w	g	f	e	e	x	o	d	a	d	e	k	k
u	w	j	k	h	q	d	h	l	c	g	l	f	j
q	q	i	o	s	p	j	q	h	l	s	c	m	g
b	a	a	d	w	o	l	d	a	a	t	q	h	l
l	l	v	q	a	b	f	l	c	e	v	b	l	k
o	e	a	w	r	r	e	y	i	n	m	e	f	s
k	m	w	d	d	y	r	p	x	i	x	d	b	f
h	z	g	o	d	d	p	p	g	r	d	p	x	v
d	w	v	x	b	e	n	a	t	e	o	a	v	r
g	p	c	z	f	l	r	p	p	p	o	n	a	h
t	n	e	n	i	t	n	o	c	n	i	s	w	m
b	d	t	u	s	r	t	a	n	w	m	g	y	s

1. When people cannot control the muscles of the bowel or bladder, they are said to be _____.

2. A _____ placed over a protective sheet can help

absorb moisture and protect the client's skin from the rubber or plastic.

3. Clients who are incontinent need to be kept _____, _____, and free from odor.

4. Offer incontinent clients a _____ frequently.

5. Bathing and good _____ help keep urine and feces from irritating the skin.

6. Clients who have lost _____ or _____ control need reassurance and understanding.

12. Explain the guidelines for assisting with bowel or bladder retraining

Fill in the Blank.

1. Encourage the client to eat foods that are high in _____.

2. Wear _____ when handling body wastes.

3. Encourage the client to drink plenty of _____. Do this even if urinary incontinence is a problem.

4. Never show _____ or _____ toward clients who are incontinent. The problem is out of their control.

5. Offer _____ words for successes or even attempts to control bladder and bowels.

6. Do not _____ the client.

7. Assist your client with good _____. This prevents skin breakdown and promotes proper hygiene.

13. Describe the benefits of deep breathing exercises

Short Answer.

What can deep breathing exercises help?

_____
_____
_____
_____
_____
_____
_____
_____

16

Medications and Technology in Home Care

1. List four guidelines for safe and proper use of medications

True or False.

Mark each statement with either a "T" for true or an "F" for false.

1. _____ Home health aides must never handle or administer medications unless specifically trained and assigned to do so.

2. _____ Home health aides are not allowed to touch the client's medication containers in any way.

3. _____ It is not important for the home health aide to know what medications the client is taking.

4. _____ Home health aides should report any symptoms, such as dizziness, stomachache, or vomiting, because these could indicate a side effect or drug interaction.

5. _____ Aspirin and ibuprofen are examples of over-the-counter drugs.

2. Identify the five "rights" of medications

Word Search.

List each of the five "rights" of medications below, and then find them in the word search.

1. The right _____
2. The right _____
3. The right _____
4. The right _____
5. The right _____

e	b	g	q	k	d	x	m	c	q	r	w	u	k
i	f	a	c	i	i	m	e	h	d	z	t	v	q
g	n	t	o	n	o	f	d	t	l	i	t	b	i
t	c	x	p	u	j	j	i	u	m	v	n	k	m
o	l	d	g	w	z	p	c	e	b	f	r	j	h
b	i	u	k	g	g	f	a	j	y	q	z	k	c
u	e	c	w	o	w	j	t	q	x	e	q	j	d
l	n	j	f	w	p	c	i	s	q	x	p	w	k
g	t	a	p	m	l	h	o	a	m	o	u	n	t
i	p	f	y	z	e	b	n	r	a	y	q	t	t
t	f	i	h	q	l	f	b	e	o	k	v	f	c
t	n	w	a	m	e	w	p	k	t	u	n	v	i
i	x	q	i	h	d	r	g	v	c	l	t	i	n
f	p	m	l	t	o	i	e	b	g	t	n	e	w

3. Explain how to assist a client with self-administered medications

True or False.

Mark each statement with either a "T" for true or an "F" for false.

1. _____ All medications should be taken with food to avoid stomach irritation.

2. _____ To avoid any problems with drug interactions, you should document every medication the client takes, whether it is part of the treatment plan or not.

3. _____ Sedatives should never be mixed with alcohol.

4. _____ You can remind a client when it is time to take medication.

5. _____ Allergic reactions to medication may require emergency intervention.

4. Identify observations about medications that should be reported right away

Short Answer.

1. What should you do if your client shows signs of a reaction to a medication or complains of side effects?

   _____
   _____
   _____

2. What should you do if your client takes medication in the wrong amount, at the wrong time, or takes the wrong kind of medication?

   _____
   _____
   _____

5. Describe what to do in an emergency involving medications

Scenarios.

1. Mrs. Mallory takes several prescription medications each day as ordered by her physician. On the day you are scheduled to visit her, you arrive at her home to find Mrs. Mallory sitting down in a chair and looking very ill. When you ask her if she is okay, she tells you that she feels very sick to her stomach and she thinks she might faint. Mrs. Mallory says that she might have taken too much medication, because she couldn't remember if she had already taken her morning dosage. What should you do?

   _____
   _____
   _____
   _____
   _____
   _____

2. You arrive at Mr. MacIntyre's home at 8:30 a.m. and find him lying in bed. You are unable to wake him, and then you notice several bottles of pills on the table next to the bed. They are all open, and some of the pills are scattered on the table and the floor. What do you do?

   _____
   _____
   _____
   _____
   _____
   _____
   _____
   _____

6. Identify methods of medication storage

True or False.

Mark each statement with either a "T" for true or an "F" for false.

1. _____ The client's medication should be kept separate from medicine used by other members of the household.

2. _____ If young children or confused adults are present in the home, medications should be stored on top of the refrigerator where they cannot be reached.

3. _____ Store all medications away from heat and light, as appropriate.

4. _____ If medication has expired, you should discard it in the trash.

7. Identify signs of drug misuse and abuse and know how to report these

Multiple Choice.

Circle the letter of the answer that best completes the statement or answers the question.

1. Drug misuse and abuse includes which of the following?

   a. refusing to take medications

   b. mixing medication with alcohol

c. taking illegal drugs
   d. all of the above
   e. none of the above

2. The best thing to do if your client refuses to take medication is:
   a. push the client to take the medication, explaining that it is good for him or her
   b. try to find out why the client doesn't want to take the medication and report to the supervisor
   c. call 911 for emergency medical help
   d. all of the above
   e. none of the above

3. A common reason why people avoid taking prescribed medication is:
   a. they dislike the side effects
   b. they cannot afford the medication
   c. they have difficulty swallowing the pills
   d. all of the above
   e. none of the above

4. Signs of drug misuse or abuse include:
   a. increased appetite and weight gain
   b. unusual cheerfulness
   c. depression, moodiness, or anorexia
   d. all of the above
   e. none of the above

5. The drugs that pose the highest risk for causing drug dependency are:
   a. pain medications
   b. antihistamines (allergy medicine)
   c. tranquilizers
   d. both a and c
   e. all of the above

8. Demonstrate an understanding of oxygen equipment

Fill in the Blank.

1. Some clients with breathing difficulties may receive _____. It is more _____ than what we breathe in the air. You should never stop, adjust, or _____ oxygen for a client.

2. Some clients receive oxygen through a _____.

3. Clients who do not need concentrated oxygen all the time may use a _____ when they need oxygen.

4. Oxygen can be irritating to the nose and mouth. Wash and dry skin carefully, and provide frequent _____ care. Offer the client plenty of _____.

5. Oxygen is a highly _____ gas. This means it can very easily explode or catch fire.

9. Explain guidelines for the care of a client with an IV

Short Answer.

Briefly describe your only responsibility when caring for a client with an IV.

_____
_____
_____
_____
_____

17

Clients with Disabilities

1. Identify common causes of disabilities

Short Answer.

List six diseases and disorders that may cause disability.

_____
_____
_____
_____
_____
_____

2. Describe daily challenges a person with a disability may face

Short Answer.

List five daily challenges a person with a disability may face.

_____
_____
_____
_____
_____

3. Define terms related to disabilities and explain why they are important

Short Answer.

1. What are some terms you use to define yourself (i.e. race, sexual orientation, religion)? Why?

_____
_____
_____
_____
_____
_____

2. List a few terms that you think would be a more preferable way to refer to people with disabilities.

_____
_____
_____
_____
_____

4. Identify social and emotional needs of persons with disabilities

Fill in the Blank.

1. Basic social and emotional needs include independence, social interaction, a sense of worth, and _____.

2. Treat all clients with _____.

3. Do not push clients beyond their _____.

4. Give clients _____ to show you what they can do by themselves.

5. Explain how a disability may affect sexuality and intimacy

True or False.

Mark each statement with either a "T" for true or an "F" for false.

Name: _____

1. _____ A disabled person does not generally experience sexual desires.
2. _____ For disabled people, the ability to meet sexual needs may be limited.

6. Identify skills you have already learned that can be applied to clients with disabilities

Short Answer.

List three skills you have already learned that can be applied to working with clients with disabilities.

_____
_____
_____
_____

7. List five goals to work toward when assisting clients who have disabilities

Fill in the Blank.

1. Promote self-care and _____.
2. Assure the client's _____.
3. Promote the client's health and _____.
4. Maintain the client's _____ and self-worth.
5. Maintain the _____ of the client's household.

Short Answer.

6. Why is it a good idea to think about how you might feel if you had a disability when working with clients with disabilities?

_____
_____
_____

_____
_____
_____
_____
_____
_____
_____

8. Identify five qualities of excellent service needed by clients with disabilities

Short Answer.

List the five qualities of excellent service needed by clients with disabilities.

_____
_____
_____
_____
_____
_____
_____
_____

9. Explain how to adapt personal care procedures to meet the needs of clients with disabilities

True or False.

Mark each statement with either a "T" for true or an "F" for false.

1. _____ When dealing with a blind client, identify yourself immediately when you enter a room.
2. _____ Avoid touching people with cerebral palsy.
3. _____ Usually people with ALS eventually have to breathe and be fed with the assistance of ventilators and tubes.
4. _____ Quadriplegia refers to the loss of function of the muscles in arms, chest, and lower body.
5. _____ Symptoms of MS include blurred vision, tremors, poor balance, and difficulty walking.

77

6. ____ When dealing with hearing impaired clients, it is easier if you pretend you understand what they are saying even if you do not.

7. ____ Multiple sclerosis is usually not diagnosed until late adulthood.

8. ____ People with muscular dystrophy do not live past childhood.

9. ____ A person with Parkinson's disease is at a high risk for falls.

10. ____ Activities that require excessive effort should not be pursued by people who have cerebral palsy.

11. ____ Children who have Down syndrome do not appear physically different from any other child.

12. ____ Head injuries may cause paresis, which means that the entire body is affected.

13. ____ Spina bifida cannot cause brain damage.

14. ____ Rehabilitation is not necessary for clients with spinal cord injuries.

15. ____ Disabilities caused by ALS or Lou Gehrig's disease begin with muscle weakness in the limbs or throat.

16. ____ Signs of hearing loss include speaking loudly and responding inappropriately.

17. ____ Speech impairment is one effect of cerebral palsy.

18. ____ A person with Parkinson's disease may have tremors or shaking. This makes it very difficult for him or her to perform ADLs such as eating and bathing.

19. ____ You may be trained to help clients in using a prosthesis when they've had a body part amputated.

20. ____ Cataracts can be corrected with surgery.

21. ____ Emotional support is a very important part of rehabilitation for a head or spinal cord injury.

22. ____ It is a good idea to use an imaginary clock when explaining the position of objects to a visually impaired client.

23. ____ It is possible that some babies born with spina bifida will be able to walk and experience no lasting disabilities.

24. ____ Braille is a fast and easy-to-learn method for blind clients to communicate.

25. ____ Phantom sensation after an amputation is not real. Ignore clients if they mention it.

26. ____ Glaucoma is a cause of blindness.

27. ____ When dealing with a hearing impaired client, you should shout to be heard.

10. List important changes to report and document for a client with disabilities

Short Answer.

1. What should you do if you notice a client is unable to perform a task that he or she was previously able to do?

   _____
   _____
   _____
   _____

2. Give two examples of emotional changes that should be observed and reported.

   _____
   _____
   _____
   _____

Name: _____

18

Mental Health and Mental Illness

1. Identify five characteristics of mental health

Short Answer.

1. Define mental health.
   _____
   _____
   _____
   _____
   _____

2. List five characteristics of a person who is mentally healthy.
   _____
   _____
   _____
   _____
   _____
   _____
   _____
   _____
   _____
   _____

2. Identify four causes of mental illness

True or False.

Mark each statement with either a "T" for true or an "F" for false.

1. _____ Signs and symptoms of mental illness include confusion, disorientation, agitation, and anxiety.

2. _____ A situation response may be triggered by severe changes in the environment.

3. _____ A mentally healthy person cannot experience a situation response.

4. _____ Mental illness can be brought on by substance abuse or a chemical imbalance.

5. _____ The building blocks of mental health are self-respect and self-worth.

6. _____ Traumatic experiences early in life do not cause mental illness.

7. _____ Mental illness cannot be inherited.

8. _____ Extreme stress may result in mental illness.

3. Distinguish between fact and fallacy concerning mental illness

True or False.

Mark each statement with either a "T" for true or an "F" for false.

1. _____ A fallacy is a false belief.

2. _____ People who are mentally ill have the power to control their illness.

3. _____ People who are mentally ill do not want to get well.

4. _____ Mental illness is a disease just like any physical illness.

5. _____ People who are mentally ill often cannot control their emotions or responses to people and situations.

4. Explain the connection between mental and physical wellness

Short Answer.

Briefly describe why mental health is important to physical health.

_____
_____

_____
_____
_____
_____

5. List guidelines for communicating with mentally ill clients

Labeling.

Fill in the blanks to show how to practice good communication skills with mentally ill clients.

1. Stand or sit with a posture that says you're _____
2. Practice _____
3. Maintain _____ contact
4. Maintain an appropriate _____

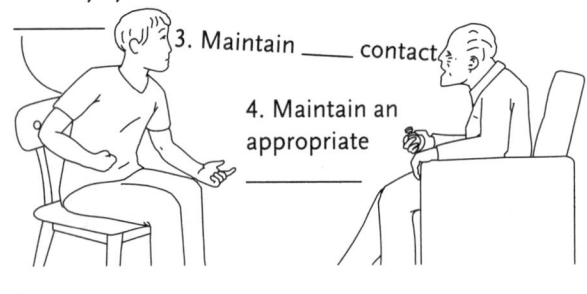

1. _____
2. _____
3. _____
4. _____

6. Identify and define common defense mechanisms

Multiple Choice.

Circle the letter of the answer that best completes the statement or answers the question.

1. Which of the following is true about defense mechanisms?
   a. They help to release tension.
   b. They help a person cope with stress.
   c. People who are mentally ill use them to a greater degree than people who are not.
   d. all of the above
   e. none of the above

2. Telling your co-worker "Let's throw spitballs at our boss" is an example of which kind of defense mechanism?
   a. displacement
   b. regression
   c. rationalization
   d. projection

3. A co-worker gets the promotion that you have wanted for a long time. When your friend asks you if you're upset, you say, "No, not at all." This is an example of:
   a. denial
   b. displacement
   c. regression
   d. projection

7. Describe the symptoms of anxiety, depression, and schizophrenia

Fill in the Blank.

Using the words below, complete each of the following statements. Each word is used only once.

anxiety	major
apathy	manic
claustrophobia	obsessive compulsive
delusions	phobia
hallucinations	schizophrenia

1. Lack of interest in activities is called _____.

2. An intense form of anxiety, such as fear of flying, is called a _____.

3. Illusions that a person sees or hears are called _____.

4. When a person washes his hands over and over again as a way of dealing with guilt, this type of behavior is called _____ disorder.

5. _____ is uneasiness or fear, often about a situation or condition.

6. _____ depression may cause a person to lose interest in everything he once cared about.

Name: _____

7. Fear of being in a confined space, such as an elevator, is called _____.

8. _____ is a brain disorder that affects a person's ability to think and communicate clearly.

9. _____ depression causes a person to swing from profound depression to extreme activity.

10. _____ are persistent false beliefs, such as thinking that other people can read one's mind.

8. Explain how medications can help a client who is mentally ill

True or False.

Mark each statement with either a "T" for true or an "F" for false.

1. _____ Mental illness cannot be treated.
2. _____ Medication and psychotherapy are commonly used to treat mental illness.
3. _____ You will be responsible for giving mentally ill clients their medication.
4. _____ Medication can allow the mentally ill to function more completely.

9. Explain your role in caring for clients who are mentally ill

Short Answer.

List four special responsibilities that you will have when caring for mentally ill clients.

_____
_____
_____
_____
_____

10. Identify important observations that should be made and reported

True or False.

Mark each statement with either a "T" for true or an "F" for false.

1. _____ It is important to report to your supervisor if a mentally ill client stops taking medication.
2. _____ You don't need to worry about a mentally ill client discussing suicide if he or she is just joking about it.
3. _____ You should report to your supervisor if a mentally ill client has an extremely happy reaction to bad news.

11. List the signs of substance abuse

Multiple Choice.

Circle the letter of the answer that best completes the statement or question.

1. Circle all of the following substances that can be abused:
   a. alcohol
   b. cigarettes
   c. decongestants
   d. diet aids
   e. illegal drugs
   f. glue
   g. paint
   h. prescription medicine

2. Your client has been acting a little strangely lately. She gets upset very easily and her eyes are always red. She does not eat much, and sometimes you can smell alcohol on her breath, even in the morning. What should you do?
   a. confront your client about what you have noticed
   b. call Alcoholics Anonymous
   c. document your observations and report them to your supervisor
   d. all of the above
   e. none of the above

19

New Mothers, Infants and Children

1. Explain the growth of home care for new mothers and infants

True or False.

Mark each statement with either a "T" for true or an "F" for false.

1. _____ Most new mothers stay in the hospital for several days to a week after childbirth.

2. _____ Bed rest is ordered if a woman shows signs of early labor.

3. _____ Home care aides are called upon to help when an expectant mother is put on bed rest by her doctor.

4. _____ New mothers today are generally more energetic when they come home than women in the past.

5. _____ Bed rest may help prevent labor from starting before the baby is ready to be born.

6. _____ Natural childbirth has been increasing in popularity.

2. Identify common neonatal disorders

Short Answer.

List three common neonatal disorders.

_____
_____
_____
_____
_____

3. Identify ways of assisting a new mother with her transition to the home

Fill in the Blank.

Use this list of words and phrases to fill in the blanks in the following sentences.

caesarean section   housekeeping
care plan   monitor
diapering   support
episiotomy   bathing
feeding

1. An incision sometimes made in the perineal area during vaginal delivery is an _____.

2. Since each situation is different, what you do to care for the new mother will be spelled out in the _____.

3. Basic care for the baby includes _____, _____, and _____.

4. You may be required to do light _____ to help the new mother.

5. A birthing procedure in which the baby is delivered through an incision in the mother's abdomen is called a _____.

6. You may be asked to _____ the equipment if the baby is receiving oxygen.

7. More care may be required depending on how much _____ the mother has from her family or others.

Name: _____

83

4. List important observations to report and document

Short Answer.

Document the following scenario.

You arrive at your client's house at 8 a.m. to care for baby Eric, a two-day-old newborn, and find the house dirty, the new mother Anne in a sitz bath, and baby Eric in the crib crying. The mother is also crying and complains of getting "no sleep last night." What course of action should you take? How would you document this?

_____
_____
_____
_____
_____
_____
_____
_____
_____
_____
_____
_____

5. Explain guidelines for safely handling a baby

Labeling.

Label the type of hold shown in each figure.

1. _____

2. _____

3. _____

6. Describe guidelines for assisting with feeding a baby

Multiple Choice.

Circle the letter of the answer that best completes the statement or answers the question.

1. If the baby does not latch onto the nipple right away, the mother should stroke his:
   a. toes
   b. elbows
   c. cheek
   d. forehead
   e. none of the above

2. Many professionals recommend that mothers try breastfeeding for _____ week(s) before deciding whether to continue or stop.
   a. five
   b. ten
   c. one
   d. two
   e. none of the above

84

3. Powdered formula is sold in:
   a. bottles
   b. one- or two-pound cans
   c. sterilized pitchers
   d. covered plastic bowls
   e. none of the above

4. The cheapest formula is usually:
   a. ready-to-feed
   b. concentrated liquid
   c. powdered
   d. prepared
   e. none of the above

5. A good position for breastfeeding is:
   a. lying face down on the bed
   b. sitting upright in a comfortable chair
   c. rocking rapidly in a chair
   d. bending over the crib
   e. none of the above

6. What food should the mother not eat because it affects breast milk?
   a. chocolate
   b. fruit
   c. yogurt
   d. fish
   e. none of the above

7. Before feeding, check the temperature of the formula on your wrist. It should feel:
   a. warm
   b. hot
   c. cold
   d. frozen
   e. none of the above

8. The mother can break the suction of a nursing baby by:
   a. pulling down the baby's ears
   b. putting her finger in the baby's mouth
   c. sucking on the baby's toes
   d. shaking the baby
   e. none of the above

7. Explain guidelines for bathing and changing a baby

True or False.

Mark each statement with either a "T" for true or an "F" for false.

1. _____ You should wear disposable gloves when changing or bathing a baby.
2. _____ You should dry a baby's head immediately after washing his hair.
3. _____ Test a baby's bath temperature by dipping the baby's hand in it to see if it turns red.
4. _____ Moisture contributes to diaper rash.
5. _____ It is okay to have both hands off the baby if it's only for a minute.
6. _____ Children generally wear diapers until they are 8 to 12 months old.
7. _____ Newborns will need between six and ten diaper changes in 24 hours.
8. _____ Always use baby powder after giving a baby a bath.
9. _____ If a newborn baby has a loose bowel movement with every feeding, you should be concerned.
10. _____ Babies should be changed frequently to avoid diaper rash.

8. Explain guidelines for special care

Matching.

For each of the following terms, write the letter of the correct definition from the list below.

1. _____ apnea
2. _____ circumcision
3. _____ oxygen
4. _____ rubbing alcohol
5. _____ umbilical cord

a. The cord that connects the baby to the placenta

Name: _____

b. Used for care of the umbilical cord stump to prevent infection

c. Given to some babies who have breathing problems; it is extremely flammable

d. The removal of part of the foreskin of the penis

e. The state of not breathing

9. Identify special physical, mental, and emotional needs of children

Short Answer.

1. List some examples of physical needs that children have.

   _____
   _____
   _____
   _____
   _____

2. List an example of a mental need that children have.

   _____
   _____
   _____

3. List some examples of emotional needs that children have.

   _____
   _____
   _____
   _____
   _____
   _____

10. List symptoms of common childhood illnesses and the required care

Fill in the Blank.

1. Cleaning, disinfection, and _____ are the best ways to control infection.

2. Infant acetaminophen is _____ than children's acetaminophen, and the dosage is much smaller.

3. Frequent loose or watery bowel movements are called _____.

4. Children with diarrhea may experience _____, thus doctors may recommend electrolyte-replacement drinks.

5. In general, children should not be given _____, because it has been associated with some serious disorders.

6. The BRAT diet consists of bananas, rice, applesauce, and _____.

7. Treatment of a fever includes a lukewarm bath or _____.

8. _____ foods, such as pasta or crackers are usually allowed when children have diarrhea.

9. Rest and _____ are recommended for fevers.

10. Too much acetaminophen can cause _____ damage.

11. Identify guidelines for working with children

Scenarios.

Read the following scenarios and decide how to respond.

1. Patrick and his older brother Greg have just returned home from school. Patrick is upset because he did not win a prize for his science project, but his brother did. He cried at school, and some of the other kids made fun of him. He becomes visibly distressed again as he relates this story to you. How can you respond to Patrick?

   _____
   _____

Name: _____

3. Child neglect is:

2. You notice that Doug has been withdrawn all afternoon. He didn't go outside to play after school, and at dinner, he refuses to eat anything. He makes a couple of comments, such as "nobody cares about me." What are some things you can do?

12. List the signs of child abuse and neglect and know how to report them

Short Answer.

1. Psychological abuse includes:

2. Sexual abuse includes:

20

Common Chronic and Acute Conditions

1. Define arthritis and identify treatments and care guidelines

Short Answer.

1. What does arthritis mean?
   _____
   _____
   _____

2. List five common treatments for arthritis.
   _____
   _____
   _____
   _____
   _____
   _____

3. List five care guidelines for arthritis.
   _____
   _____
   _____
   _____
   _____
   _____
   _____
   _____

2. Define cancer and list eight risk factors for cancer

Fill in the Blank.

Fill in the blanks with the words listed below.

   benign   malignant
   cancer   tumor
   cure

1. _____ is a general term used to describe many types of malignant tumors.

2. A _____ is a cluster of abnormally growing cells.

3. _____ tumors grow slowly in local areas and are considered non-cancerous.

4. _____ tumors grow rapidly and invade surrounding tissues.

5. There is no known _____ for cancer.

3. List seven warning signs of cancer

Mark the American Cancer Society's seven warning signs of cancer below.

1. _____ Change in bowel or bladder habits
2. _____ Difficulty breathing
3. _____ Dizziness
4. _____ Thickening or lump in breast
5. _____ Memory loss
6. _____ Obvious change in wart or mole
7. _____ Pain or swelling of the joints
8. _____ Persistent hoarseness or nagging cough
9. _____ Persistent indigestion or difficulty swallowing
10. _____ Nausea or vomiting
11. _____ Sweet, fruity breath odor
12. _____ Sore that does not heal
13. _____ Unusual bleeding or discharge from body opening
14. _____ Headache

4. Identify common treatments for cancer

Multiple Choice.

Circle the letter of the answer that best completes the statement or answers the question.

1. The key treatment for malignant tumors of the skin, breast, bladder, colon, rectum, stomach, and muscle is:
    a. surgery
    b. chemotherapy
    c. radiation
    d. diet and exercise
    e. none of the above

2. Nausea, vomiting, diarrhea, hair loss, and decreased resistance to infection are all side effects of which treatment?
    a. surgery
    b. chemotherapy
    c. radiation
    d. both b and c
    e. none of the above

3. This treatment method uses drugs to destroy cancer cells and limit the rate of cell growth:
    a. surgery
    b. chemotherapy
    c. radiation
    d. all of the above
    e. none of the above

4. This treatment method involves removing as much of the tumor as possible to prevent cancer from spreading:
    a. surgery
    b. chemotherapy
    c. radiation
    d. all of the above
    e. none of the above

5. This treatment method kills normal and abnormal cells in a limited area, sometimes causing skin to become sore, irritated, or burned.
    a. surgery
    b. chemotherapy
    c. radiation
    d. all of the above
    e. none of the above

5. Describe care guidelines for the client who has cancer

Multiple Choice.

Circle the letter of the answer that best completes the statement or answers the question.

1. To help promote good nutrition, you can do the following:
    a. serve meals four to six times a day
    b. serve favorite foods that are high in nutrition
    c. serve liquid nutritional supplements in addition to meals
    d. all of the above
    e. none of the above

2. If your client is experiencing pain, you should:
    a. assist with comfort measures
    b. report to your supervisor
    c. give the client pain medication
    d. both a and b
    e. all of the above

3. In providing skin care, which of the following is NOT a good idea?
    a. use lotion regularly on dry or delicate skin
    b. avoid moving client unless absolutely necessary
    c. offer back rubs for comfort and circulation
    d. all of the above
    e. none of the above

Name: _____

4. Which of the following is NOT a good idea when providing good oral care?
   a. rinsing with commercial mouthwash
   b. using a soft-bristled toothbrush
   c. assisting client to brush and floss regularly
   d. all of the above
   e. none of the above

5. Which of the following is a good idea for communicating with a client who has cancer?
   a. Insist that the client tell you what he or she is going through.
   b. Listen to the client if he or she feels like talking.
   c. If the client is worried, tell him or her "It'll all be fine."
   d. all of the above
   e. none of the above

6. You are caring for Mrs. Brady, a client who has cancer. Mrs. Brady has a lot of visitors, and most of them call before they come over. One visitor has a habit of stopping by whenever she happens to be in the area, and today she has come at a very bad time for Mrs. Brady. What should you tell this visitor?
   a. Mrs. Brady enjoys your visits, but unfortunately this is not a good time for her. Perhaps you can give her a phone call later on. I'll certainly let her know you were here.
   b. Mrs. Brady can't just drop whatever she is doing to entertain you. You should call before you come over.
   c. Most people know that it is very inconsiderate to stop by someone's house without calling first.
   d. Mrs. Brady is having a bath right now. You should stop by later.
   e. Lady, I'm just the caregiver. It's not my fault if Mrs. Brady doesn't want to see you.

6. Identify community resources available to people with cancer and their families

Short Answer.

List three types of organizations that provide services and support for people with cancer and their families.

_____
_____
_____
_____
_____

7. Describe diabetes and identify its signs and complications

Short Answer.

1. What causes diabetes?

_____
_____
_____
_____
_____

2. List three signs and symptoms of diabetes.

_____
_____
_____
_____

Multiple Choice.

Circle the letter of the answer that best completes the statement.

3. Diabetes can lead to the following complications:
   a. changes in the circulatory system
   b. damage to the eyes
   c. impaired wound healing
   d. all of the above
   e. none of the above

4. Changes in the circulatory system can cause:
   a. kidney and nerve damage
   b. hair loss
   c. opportunistic infections
   d. all of the above
   e. none of the above

5. Damage to the eyes can cause:
   a. dizziness
   b. nausea
   c. blindness
   d. all of the above
   e. none of the above

6. Poor circulation and impaired wound healing may result in:
   a. infected wounds
   b. foot ulcers
   c. gangrene
   d. all of the above
   e. none of the above

7. Gangrene can lead to:
   a. loss of bowel control
   b. amputation
   c. paralysis
   d. all of the above
   e. none of the above

8. Describe the differences between insulin shock and diabetic coma, and list care for each

Matching.

For each of the following statements, decide whether it describes insulin shock or diabetic coma. Then write "I" for insulin shock or "D" for diabetic coma.

1. _____ Also known as hypoglycemia.
2. _____ Also known as hyperglycemia.
3. _____ Can result from too much food.
4. _____ Can result from too little food.
5. _____ Dry skin is a sign of this.
6. _____ Perspiration is a sign of this.
7. _____ Blurred vision is a sign of this.
8. _____ Flushed cheeks are a sign of this.
9. _____ Nausea and vomiting are a sign of this.
10. _____ Abdominal pain is a sign of this.
11. _____ Numbness of the lips and tongue is a sign of this.
12. _____ Confusion is a sign of this.
13. _____ Sweet, fruity breath odor is a sign of this.
14. _____ Cold, clammy skin is a sign of this.

9. List care guidelines for the client with diabetes

True or False.

Mark each statement with either a "T" for true or an "F" for false.

1. _____ Meals must be eaten at the same time every day for the client with diabetes.
2. _____ If your client is not following her diet, report this to your supervisor.
3. _____ Encourage the client with diabetes to eat as many carbohydrates as possible.
4. _____ Exercise has not been shown to help clients with diabetes.
5. _____ Home care aides are not permitted to inject insulin.
6. _____ Check the expiration date on insulin before giving it to the client.
7. _____ All states require that home health aides test a diabetic client's blood and urine every day for sugar or insulin levels.
8. _____ A small sore on a diabetic client can be dangerous.

Name: _____

91

9. _____ Home health aides should never cut any client's toenails, but especially not a diabetic client's toenails.

10. _____ Diabetics should go barefoot.

10. Describe a meal plan for the client with diabetes

Short Answer.

Design a sample meal plan that follows the Sample Meal Plan on page 275 in the textbook and uses foods from the Exchange List Sample Items, also in the same box.

Breakfast:

_____
_____
_____

Snack:

_____
_____
_____

Lunch:

_____
_____
_____

Snack:

_____
_____
_____

Dinner:

_____
_____
_____

Snack:

_____
_____
_____

11. Define cerebral vascular accident (CVA) and list common warning signs

Crossword.

Across

1. _____ is weakness on one side of the body.

4. A warning sign of a CVA is _____.

6. It is the result of a lack of _____ in the brain.

7. A stroke is caused when the blood supply to the brain is cut off suddenly by a _____ or a ruptured blood vessel.

Down

2. _____ is the inability to speak or to speak clearly.

3. Another name for cerebral vascular accident is a _____.

5. _____ is paralysis on one side of the body.

12. Describe six common physical changes in CVA clients

Mark an "X" next to the physical changes listed below that a client who has had a stroke may experience.

1. _____ confusion
2. _____ decreased circulation
3. _____ developing pressure sores
4. _____ difficulty speaking
5. _____ difficulty breathing
6. _____ difficulty swallowing
7. _____ hallucinations or delusions
8. _____ inability to speak
9. _____ increased thirst and hunger
10. _____ loss of sensations such as temperature or touch
11. _____ loss of cognitive abilities
12. _____ loss of bowel or bladder control
13. _____ memory loss
14. _____ night sweats
15. _____ persistent hoarseness or a nagging cough
16. _____ poor judgment
17. _____ restlessness
18. _____ tendency to ignore one side of the body
19. _____ wandering
20. _____ weakness on one side of the body

13. Describe care guidelines and communication techniques for the CVA client

True or False.

Mark each statement with either a "T" for true or an "F" for false.

1. _____ Clients with paralysis or loss of movement do not need physical therapy.
2. _____ Range-of-motion exercises strengthen muscles and keep joints mobile.
3. _____ Leg exercises improve circulation.
4. _____ When helping with transfers or ambulation, stand on the client's stronger side.
5. _____ Always use a gait belt for safety.
6. _____ Refer to the side that has been affected by stroke as the "bad" side.
7. _____ Gestures and facial expressions are important in communicating with the CVA client.
8. _____ Clients who suffer confusion or memory loss due to a stroke may feel more secure if you establish a routine of care.
9. _____ CVA clients are not at risk of falling.
10. _____ Clients with a loss of sensation could easily burn themselves.
11. _____ For safety purposes, unnecessary clutter and throw rugs should be removed.
12. _____ Pay close attention to changes in the skin of the CVA client, and observe for skin breakdown.
13. _____ Let the client do things for him- or herself whenever possible.

Scenarios.

Read each of the following statements, and answer the questions.

14. Jody, a home health aide, is getting ready to prepare lunch for Mr. Elliot, who is recovering from a stroke. Mr. Elliot has difficulty communicating and also suffers from confusion. "Let's see," Jody says. "For lunch we can have soup, sandwiches, some leftover

Name: _____

93

casserole, or I can make a salad. Now, what would you like to eat?" What is wrong with the way Jody is communicating with Mr. Elliot?

_____
_____
_____
_____
_____
_____
_____

15. Mr. Elliot's wife comes home after running some errands and asks how her husband is doing. As she and Jody walk into the kitchen where Mr. Elliot is sitting, Jody says, "Mr. Elliot is having trouble today with his eating. Just look at him. He's spilled all over himself." What is wrong with what Jody has just said?

_____
_____
_____
_____
_____
_____

16. Jody notices that Mr. Elliot seems to be having trouble saying words clearly. He is beginning to get frustrated because he can't tell Jody what he wants. Jody decides to ask only yes or no questions, so she tells Mr. Elliot, "If you find it too difficult to speak right now, why don't you try nodding your head for "yes" and shaking your head for "no"." What is Jody doing right?

_____
_____
_____
_____
_____
_____
_____

Fill in the Blank.

17. When assisting with a transfer for a client with one-sided weakness, always lead with the _____ side.

18. Dress the _____ side first. This prevents unnecessary bending.

19. Undress the _____ side first.

20. _____ equipment is used to help the client dress himself.

21. When assisting a CVA client to eat, place the food in the client's _____

14. Identify common circulatory disorders, their symptoms, and care guidelines

Matching.

For each of the following terms, write the letter of the correct definition from the list below.

1. _____ angina pectoris
2. _____ atherosclerosis
3. _____ congestive heart failure
4. _____ diuretics
5. _____ dyspnea
6. _____ hypertension
7. _____ myocardial infarction
8. _____ nitroglycerin

a. difficulty breathing

b. the condition in which the heart fails to pump effectively, causing blood to back up into the heart instead of circulating

c. another name for chest pain

d. another name for high blood pressure

e. medication that relaxes the walls of the coronary arteries

f. a condition in which blood flow to the heart muscle is completely blocked and the muscle cell dies

g. drugs that reduce fluid in the body

h. a hardening and narrowing of the blood vessels

15. Define COPD and list care guidelines

Multiple Choice.

Circle the letter of the answer that best completes the statement.

1. Clients with COPD have difficulty with this:
   a. breathing
   b. urination
   c. maintaining weight
   d. vision

2. A constant fear of a person who has COPD is:
   a. constipation
   b. incontinence
   c. not being able to breathe
   d. heart attack

3. Clients who have COPD may experience the following:
   a. poor appetite
   b. lack of sleep
   c. fear of suffocation
   d. all of the above

4. A client with COPD should be positioned:
   a. lying flat on his back
   b. sitting upright
   c. lying on his stomach
   d. lying on his side

5. Your role in caring for a client with COPD includes:
   a. being calm and supportive
   b. encouraging independence with ADLs
   c. practicing good infection control
   d. all of the above

16. Define HIV and AIDS and describe care guidelines

True or False.

Mark each statement with either a "T" for true or an "F" for false.

1. _____ HIV and AIDS are the same thing.

2. _____ HIV can only be transmitted sexually.

3. _____ The first stage of HIV infection involves symptoms similar to flu.

4. _____ There is no known cure for AIDS.

5. _____ AIDS dementia complex occurs in the early stages of AIDS.

Short Answer.

6. List five signs and symptoms of HIV infection and AIDS.

   _____
   _____
   _____
   _____
   _____

7. What is an opportunistic infection?

   _____
   _____
   _____
   _____
   _____

Multiple Choice.

Circle the letter of the answer that best completes the statement.

Name: _____

8. Care for the person with AIDS should focus on:
   a. helping to find a cure for HIV
   b. preventing visits from friends and family
   c. providing relief of symptoms and preventing complications
   d. all of the above
   e. none of the above

9. If your AIDS client has a poor appetite, you should:
   a. help them to relax before meals
   b. serve familiar and favorite foods
   c. report appetite loss to your supervisor
   d. all of the above
   e. none of the above

10. It is extremely important to follow safety guidelines when preparing food for the person with AIDS, because:
    a. food-borne illnesses can cause death
    b. you might become infected with HIV
    c. you might infect family members with HIV
    d. all of the above
    e. none of the above

11. While preparing food for the person with AIDS, you must:
    a. wash your hands frequently
    b. keep all utensils, counter tops, and cutting boards clean
    c. wash and cook foods thoroughly
    d. all of the above
    e. none of the above

12. AIDS clients who have infections of the mouth and esophagus may need to eat food that is:
    a. spicy
    b. low in acid
    c. dry
    d. all of the above
    e. none of the above

13. Painful sores in the mouth may be relieved by:
    a. drinking orange juice
    b. rubbing with a soft toothbrush
    c. rinsing frequently with warm salt water
    d. all of the above
    e. none of the above

14. Someone who has nausea and vomiting should:
    a. eat small frequent meals
    b. avoid high-fat and spicy foods
    c. drink liquids and eat salty foods
    d. all of the above
    e. none of the above

15. The "BRAT" diet is helpful for:
    a. diarrhea
    b. weight gain
    c. nausea and vomiting
    d. all of the above
    e. none of the above

16. Fluids are important for clients who have diarrhea because:
    a. diarrhea rapidly depletes the body of fluids
    b. diarrhea can be prevented by drinking a lot of fluids
    c. diarrhea is an infection that can be flushed out by fluids
    d. all of the above
    e. none of the above

17. The following is helpful in dealing with neuropathy:
    a. pain medications
    b. wearing loose, soft slippers
    c. using a bed cradle
    d. all of the above
    e. none of the above

18. People with AIDS often suffer from anxiety and depression because:
    a. AIDS is incurable.
    b. Others may have negative attitudes about people with AIDS.
    c. They may have already lost friends and family members to the disease.
    d. all of the above
    e. none of the above

17. Describe normal changes of aging in the brain

Multiple Choice.

Circle the letter of the answer that best completes the statement.

1. The ability to think logically and quickly is called:
    a. cognition
    b. dementia
    c. awareness
    d. all of the above
    e. none of the above

2. Cognitive impairment affects:
    a. social security reform
    b. motor skills
    c. concentration and memory
    d. all of the above
    e. none of the above

3. Home health aides can help elderly clients by:
    a. doing as much as possible for them
    b. encouraging them to make lists of things to remember
    c. reminding them every time they forget something
    d. all of the above
    e. none of the above

18. Define dementia and recognize its causes

True or False.

Mark each statement with either a "T" for true or an "F" for false.

1. ____ Dementia is the loss of mental abilities such as thinking, remembering, reasoning, and communicating.

2. ____ Dementia is a normal part of aging.

19. Describe Alzheimer's disease and identify its stages and related behaviors

True or False.

Mark each statement with either a "T" for true or an "F" for false.

1. ____ Alzheimer's disease begins with forgetfulness and confusion and progresses to complete loss of all ability to care for oneself.

2. ____ Different people with Alzheimer's disease may show different symptoms at different times.

3. ____ A home health aide should perform as many activities as possible for clients with Alzheimer's disease.

4. ____ Alzheimer's disease cannot be cured.

20. Identify personal attitudes helpful in caring for people with AD or any dementia

Short Answer.

For each of the following personal attitudes in caring for Alzheimer's clients, briefly describe why each attitude is helpful.

1. Don't take it personally. Why?

_____

_____

_____

_____

Name: _____

97

2. Put yourself in their shoes. Why?
_____
_____
_____
_____
_____
_____

3. Work with the symptoms and behaviors you see. Why?
_____
_____
_____
_____
_____
_____

4. Work as a team. Why?
_____
_____
_____
_____
_____
_____

5. Take care of yourself. Why?
_____
_____
_____
_____
_____
_____

6. Work with family members. Why?
_____
_____
_____
_____
_____

7. Remember the goals of the client care plan. Why?
_____
_____
_____
_____
_____
_____

21. List three strategies for better communication with Alzheimer's clients

True or False.

Mark each statement with either a "T" for true or an "F" for false.

1. _____ When communicating with an Alzheimer's client, speak in a calm, quiet manner.

2. _____ Plenty of noise and distractions can help the client cope with having Alzheimer's disease.

3. _____ Perseveration means to wander constantly.

4. _____ When working with an Alzheimer's client, you may have to repeat yourself several times.

5. _____ You should always use the same words and phrases when repeating something.

6. _____ A drawing of a toilet can be a form of communication.

7. _____ Nonverbal communication is not effective when dealing with Alzheimer's clients.

22. Describe a safe environment for a client with AD

Short Answer.

1. List three things you can do to organize the home for disoriented clients.
_____
_____

98

_____
_____
_____

2. List three things you can do to organize the home for clients who wander.

_____
_____
_____
_____
_____

3. List three things you can do to organize the home for clients who pace.

_____
_____
_____

23. Explain how to assist with personal care and activities of daily living for the client with AD

For each of the following statements, write "good idea" if the statement is a good idea for clients with Alzheimer's disease, and "bad idea" if the statement is a bad idea.

1. Use nonslip mats, tub seats, and hand holds to ensure safety during bathing.
   _____

2. Always bathe the client at the same time every day, even if he or she is agitated.
   _____

3. Always use the same steps and explain what you are doing the same way every time.
   _____

4. Do not attempt to groom the client, since he or she may not enjoy this.
   _____

5. Choose clothes that are simple to put on.
   _____

6. If the client is incontinent, do not give him or her fluids.
   _____

7. Mark the restroom with a sign as a reminder of when to use it and where it is.
   _____

8. Check the skin regularly for signs of irritation.
   _____

9. Follow Standard Precautions when caring for the client.
   _____

10. Do not encourage exercise as this will make the client more agitated.
    _____

11. Serve finger foods if the client tends to wander during meals.
    _____

12. Schedule meals at the same time every day.
    _____

13. Serve new kinds of foods as often as possible to stimulate the client.
    _____

14. Offer one course at a time, using one utensil at a time.
    _____

15. Monitor weight accurately and frequently.
    _____

16. Do not encourage independence as this can lead to aggressive behavior.
    _____

17. Provide a daily calendar to encourage activities.
    _____

18. Reward positive behavior with smiles, hugs, warm touches, and thank-yous.
    _____

24. List eight difficult behaviors common in clients with AD and describe ways to manage each

Scenarios.

1. Mr. Imfeld is showing signs of agitation. Patrick, his caregiver, notices that the television in the next room is playing a very loud commercial. What should Patrick do?

Name: _____

_____

1. Mr. Imfeld still seems agitated. What can Patrick do now?

2. Mrs. Drew is wandering around the house aimlessly. Her caregiver, Ruth, knows that she has just eaten and has gone to the restroom. Mrs. Drew had a long nap earlier. What can Ruth do about Mrs. Drew's wandering?

3. Mrs. Drew becomes extremely agitated when her new caregiver, Ruth, tries to give her a tub bath. Mrs. Drew's daughter is present and tells Ruth that her mother is used to taking showers. What can Ruth do?

4. Lately, Fran notices that Mr. Young seems withdrawn and listless (has no energy). He refuses to eat and seems to have lost all interest in his favorite activities. What can Fran do?

5. Mrs. Montoya persists in asking her caregiver, Jamie, who she is. What should Jamie do?

25. Describe creative therapies for clients with AD

Fill in the Blank.

Fill in the blanks with the words listed below.

Activity therapy   Reminiscence therapy

Reality orientation   Validation therapy

1. Encouraging the client to talk about the past and explore memories is _____.

2. Using calendars, clocks, signs, and lists to help the client remember who and where she is is called _____.

3. Using activities to prevent boredom and frustration and improve self-esteem is _____.

4. Letting the client believe he lives in the past or in imaginary circumstances, without attempting to reorient him is _____.

21

Clean, Safe and Healthy Environments

1. Describe how housekeeping affects physical and psychological well-being

Short Answer.

What are some reasons you should maintain an orderly and clean household for your client?

_____

_____

_____

_____

_____

2. List qualities needed to manage a home and describe general housekeeping guidelines

True or False.

Mark each statement with either a "T" for true or an "F" for false.

1. _____ Your primary responsibility as a home health aide is to clean your client's kitchen.

2. _____ You should expect that all members of the household will be able to help with housekeeping.

3. _____ Your assignment might include managing a client's finances.

4. _____ You may need to be flexible with regard to household maintenance.

5. _____ As a home health aide, you will never have to do a client's laundry.

6. _____ You will be solely responsible for determining which home maintenance activities you will perform.

7. _____ You should be sensitive towards your client's customs and beliefs.

8. _____ You need to use cleaning materials and methods that are acceptable to and approved by clients and their families.

9. _____ Using proper body mechanics is not important in performing housekeeping chores.

3. Describe cleaning products and equipment

True or False.

Mark each statement with either a "T" for true or an "F" for false.

1. _____ All-purpose cleaners can be used on several types of surfaces.

2. _____ It is okay to mix bleach and ammonia to clean surfaces that are really stained.

3. _____ Abrasive cleaners are used mostly for bathing clients.

4. _____ A sponge is generally used to soften and remove soil on washable surfaces.

5. _____ Vacuum cleaner bags should be checked frequently.

6. _____ Some cleaning products can cause burns.

7. _____ You can use a specialty cleaner to clean the oven.

8. _____ There are four basic types of home cleaning products available.

Name: _____   101

4. Describe proper cleaning methods for living areas, kitchens, bathrooms, and storage areas

Multiple Choice.

Circle the letter of the answer that best completes the statement or answers the question.

1. Examples of essential items which should be kept close by the client include:
   a. tissues
   b. potato chips
   c. nail polish
   d. cosmetics
   e. none of the above

2. Frequent causes of falls and accidents in the home are:
   a. well-lit hallways
   b. wet floors
   c. clean floors
   d. leftover food scraps
   e. none of the above

3. In the kitchen, diseases may be transmitted by:
   a. mops
   b. infestation
   c. contaminated food surfaces
   d. both b and c
   e. none of the above

4. It is a good idea to dust this often, unless the client has allergies:
   a. five times a week
   b. once a week
   c. once every two months
   d. twice a month
   e. none of the above

5. You can defrost a freezer quickly by:
   a. using a warm knife to chip at the ice
   b. lighting matches near the ice
   c. using a blow torch
   d. placing pans of hot water in it
   e. none of the above

6. In order to remove odors, you can use:
   a. flour
   b. baking soda
   c. sugar
   d. baking powder
   e. none of the above

7. You can sterilize dishes by:
   a. using a dishwasher
   b. using cold water
   c. using an oven cleaner
   d. drying them with a dish towel
   e. none of the above

8. How often should you dispose of garbage?
   a. daily
   b. weekly
   c. monthly
   d. bi-annually
   e. none of the above

9. Basic bathroom hygiene includes:
   a. removing hair from drain strainers
   b. placing soiled towels on the bathroom sink
   c. scrubbing the tub and shower after each use
   d. both a and c
   e. none of the above

10. Instead of glass cleaner, you can mix water and:
    a. white wine
    b. white vinegar
    c. apple juice
    d. spray starch
    e. none of the above

11. In what situation do mold and mildew grow best?
    a. in extreme cold
    b. in dry heat
    c. when it is moist and warm
    d. in frigid winds
    e. none of the above

102

12. How many parts water should you dilute bleach with to clean bathroom surfaces?
    a. twelve parts
    b. four parts
    c. one part
    d. six parts
    e. none of the above

13. Vacuum floors and rugs at least:
    a. once a month
    b. twice a week
    c. once a week
    d. once a day
    e. none of the above

5. Describe how to prepare a cleaning schedule

Create a sample cleaning schedule for an immobile client.

Immediately:

_____

_____

_____

Daily:

_____

_____

_____

_____

Weekly:

_____

_____

_____

Monthly:

_____

Name: _____

_____

_____

_____

_____

Less often:

_____

_____

_____

_____

_____

6. List special housekeeping procedures to use when infection is present

Word Search.

j	n	q	v	v	b	v	o	o	r	p	o	e	s
s	d	a	k	b	w	l	n	e	r	i	s	i	n
v	g	j	p	d	b	i	e	e	i	p	l	p	e
f	k	d	o	d	f	o	c	a	t	y	v	a	m
y	z	e	k	o	e	a	i	f	c	t	m	h	i
f	z	b	u	d	u	b	h	l	j	h	p	c	c
q	t	l	n	t	m	b	c	d	i	d	v	x	e
r	a	b	i	c	l	e	a	n	z	n	n	m	p
z	p	o	e	t	a	r	a	p	e	s	g	t	s
u	n	r	j	p	q	y	s	k	p	z	r	c	b
s	d	i	s	i	n	f	e	c	t	a	o	t	x
j	r	l	a	t	p	o	f	x	s	d	w	x	u
u	r	n	z	d	z	w	h	h	k	b	f	u	t
u	y	a	d	p	z	x	j	j	m	c	e	f	k

Complete each of the following sentences and find your answers in the word search.

1. _____ any surfaces that contact body fluids, such as a _____, urinal and toilet.

2. Frequently remove _____ containing used tissues.

3. Keep any _____ of urine or stool in double bags away from food.

Name: _____   103

4. Take special _____ in housecleaning when you know the client has a known infectious disease.

5. Use _____ dishes and utensils for the infected client.

6. Wash dishes in hot soapy water with _____, and rinse in _____ water.

7. _____ the client's bathroom daily

7. Explain how to do laundry and care for clothes

Crossword.

5. If clients can do their own mending, they may just need you to _____ a needle.

6. Liquid chlorine bleach removes stains and _____ clothing.

8. The safest temperature for most garments is _____.

10. There are three types of bleach: liquid chlorine, powdered chlorine, and _____ bleach.

11. A delicate fabric requires _____ time in the dryer.

12. Brightly colored fabrics should be washed in _____ water.

Down

1. Before washing is done, certain especially dirty or stained items should be _____.

2. Every time you use the dryer, you should clean the _____.

3. Delicate or fragile items should be washed on the _____ cycle.

6. Folding clothes immediately after they're dried reduces _____.

7. Pressing silks on the wrong side helps prevent them from becoming _____.

8. Bleach should always be diluted with _____.

9. Sturdy permanent press items and cottons can be washed on the _____ setting.

12. You should iron collars and _____ first.

8. List special laundry precautions to use when infection is present

True or False.

Mark each statement with either a "T" for true or an "F" for false.

Across

4. Whites and towels should generally be washed in _____ water.

1. _____ When handling laundry for a client who has an infectious disease, use cold water.

2. _____ You should wear gloves when doing an infectious client's laundry.

3. _____ If an infectious disease is present, do not use liquid bleach.

4. _____ Keep an infectious client's laundry separate from other family members' laundry.

5. _____ Sort an infectious client's laundry and put in plastic bags.

6. _____ Use a disinfectant in all loads.

9. List guidelines for teaching housekeeping skills to clients' family members

Scenario.

Read the following scenario and decide how to respond.

Dave, a home health aide, is explaining to Mrs. Crawford's family how to protect against infectious diseases when doing the laundry and cleaning the kitchen. He has written a long list of instructions, and when he is done explaining, two family members still seem confused about some key points. How should Dave respond in this situation?

10. List three reasons careful bedmaking is important

Short Answer.

List three reasons why careful bedmaking is important.

11. Identify hazardous household materials

Short Answer.

Identify five hazardous household materials.

22

Clients' Nutritional Needs

1. Describe the importance of good nutrition and list the six basic nutrients

Read the following sentences and mark which of the six basic nutrients it is describing. Use a "P" for proteins, "C" for carbohydrates, "F" for fats, "V" for vitamins, "M" for minerals, and "W" for water.

1. _____ Good sources of these are fish, meat, dried beans, and cheese.
2. _____ Without this, a person can only live a few days.
3. _____ These help the body store energy.
4. _____ These add flavor to food and help to absorb certain vitamins.
5. _____ Beans and rice are examples of complementary _____.
6. _____ Examples of these are butter, oil, and salad dressing.
7. _____ They are essential for tissue growth and repair.
8. _____ The body cannot produce most of these.
9. _____ These provide fiber.
10. _____ Examples of these include bread, cereal, and potatoes.
11. _____ This is the most essential nutrient for life.
12. _____ These can be classified as monounsaturated, polyunsaturated, and saturated.
13. _____ Through perspiration, this helps to maintain body temperature.
14. _____ These can be fat-soluble or water-soluble.
15. _____ One-half to two-thirds of our body weight is this.
16. _____ Iron and calcium are examples of these.

2. List the six food groups on the USDA Food Guide Pyramid

Labeling.

Looking at the Food Guide Pyramid below, fill in the six food groups and the recommended daily servings for each group.

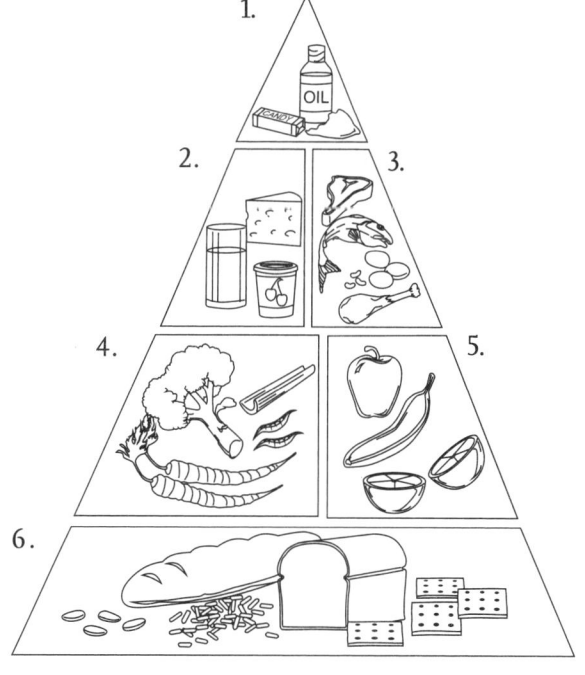

1. _____

2. _____

3. _____
_____
_____
_____

4. _____
_____
_____
_____

5. _____
_____
_____
_____

6. _____
_____
_____
_____

Short Answer.

Describe your diet during the last 24 hours and break it down into food groups and servings.

_____
_____
_____
_____
_____
_____
_____
_____

3. Identify ways to assist clients in maintaining fluid balance

True or False.

Mark each statement with either a "T" for true or an "F" for false.

1. _____ People should drink at least 1–2 glasses of water a day.

2. _____ Fluid overload occurs when the body is unable to handle the amount of fluid consumed.

3. _____ The sense of thirst diminishes in elderly people.

4. _____ People can become dehydrated by vomiting too much.

5. _____ A symptom of fluid overload is flushed, dry skin.

6. _____ In order to prevent dehydration, you should encourage clients to drink every time you see them.

7. _____ A symptom of dehydration is dark urine.

4. Identify nutritional problems of the elderly or ill

Short Answer.

1. What can unintended weight loss lead to?

_____
_____
_____

2. List five things to observe and report to your supervisor about unintended weight loss.

_____
_____
_____
_____
_____
_____

Word Search.

Complete each of the following sentences and find your answers in the word search.

3. Encourage clients to _____.

4. Provide _____ before and after meals.

5. Honor _____ likes and dislikes.

Name: _____

6. Offer many different kinds of foods and _____.

7. Allow enough _____ to finish eating.

8. Notify your supervisor if a client has trouble using _____.

9. Position clients sitting _____ for feeding.

10. If client has had a loss of _____, ask about it.

11. Record meal/snack _____.

```
e u a x w e r a c l a r o u
e k j i l n s t u m b b p s
j e a e j e t s w y e r y e
l r t t p s f l v v i g z c
q c x i n z k n e g p a p d
l j o f t i g r h p y e p o
i v p i c e a t u e s v b h
b w m v m g p c m d v a a x
j n o u e j z p l u j q l m
d o q s w f z l a o b w m w
t a t d b n t o x m e c l p
c a o o u d x g e k d m z n
e o w i x v a g c c d c i u
f u t e n s i l s i i w c t
```

Short Answer.

12. What is a nasogastric tube?

_____
_____
_____
_____

13. What is a gastrostomy?

_____
_____
_____
_____

14. What is intravenous hyperalimentation?

_____
_____
_____
_____
_____
_____
_____

5. Demonstrate awareness of regional, cultural, and religious food preferences

Short Answer.

Briefly describe some of the foods you ate while growing up. Were there any special dishes that your family made that were related to your culture, religion, or region?

_____
_____
_____
_____
_____
_____
_____
_____
_____
_____
_____
_____
_____

6. List and define common health claims on food labels

Fill in the Blank.

1. _____ meat, poultry, eggs, and dairy products come from animals that are given no antibiotics or growth hormones.

2. _____ products may contain artificial sweeteners, such as saccharin or aspartame.

107

108

3. If a product is labeled _____ or _____, it usually does not contain much fat.

4. The claims of _____, "healthy," or "good for you" may have little or no meaning.

5. Clients who must reduce their sodium or salt intake should eat foods labeled _____ or _____.

6. The best way to limit _____ is to avoid foods containing animal fats.

7. Explain the information on the FDA-required Nutrition Facts label

Multiple Choice.

Circle the letter of the answer that best completes the statement or answers the question.

1. Total calories from fat should be no more than:
   a. 30%
   b. 50%
   c. 10%
   d. 2%
   e. none of the above

2. If the percentage of daily totals for vitamins and minerals exceeds 50%, you know that:
   a. it might make you sick
   b. it is more than you need for the day
   c. it is a good source of that vitamin or mineral
   d. it should only be consumed in intervals
   e. none of the above

3. For which of the following does the FDA-required label NOT give amounts?
   a. total fat
   b. sodium
   c. calories
   d. serving size
   e. none of the above

4. The standardized nutrition label on all packaged foods is called:
   a. the label
   b. food information
   c. nutrition facts
   d. serving size information
   e. none of the above

5. The recommended daily totals are based on a _____ calorie diet.
   a. 2,500
   b. 2,000
   c. 1,000
   d. 5,000
   e. none of the above

8. Explain special or modified diets

Matching.

Read the following sentences and identify what special diet each is describing. Choose from the diets listed below.

a. Low-Sodium Diet
b. Fluid-Restricted Diet
c. Low-Protein Diet
d. Low-Fat/Low-Cholesterol Diet
e. Modified Calorie Diet
f. Dietary Management of Ulcers
g. Dietary Management of Diabetes

1. _____ To prevent further heart or kidney damage, physicians may restrict a client's fluid intake.

2. _____ In addition to restricted intake of fluids and sodium, people who have kidney disease may also be on this diet.

3. _____ People at risk for heart attacks and heart disease may be placed on these. This diet includes limiting fatty meats, egg yolks, and fried foods.

4. _____ Calories and carbohydrates must be carefully regulated in this diet. The types of foods and the amounts are

determined by the person's nutritional and energy requirements.

5. ____ Salt is restricted in this diet. Other high-sodium foods, such as ham, nuts, pickles, and canned soups, will be limited.

6. ____ Used for losing weight or preventing additional weight gain.

7. ____ This diet avoids foods that increase the levels of acid in the stomach. Alcohol, beverages containing caffeine, and spicy seasonings are some of the things that should be avoided.

Read the following meals and modify to fit the specific special diets.

8. **Regular diet**
   BREAKFAST
   Scrambled eggs
   Bacon
   Toast with butter
   Whole milk

   Low fat/cholesterol diet
   BREAKFAST

   _____

   _____

   _____

   _____

9. **Regular diet**
   LUNCH
   Ham sandwich
   Potato chips
   Canned soup
   Cookies

   Low sodium diet
   LUNCH

   _____

   _____

   _____

10. **Regular diet**
    DINNER
    Steak
    Baked potato with sour cream
    Sauteed green beans
    Chocolate cream pie

    Low fat/cholesterol diet
    DINNER

Name: _____

23

Meal Planning, Shopping, Preparation, and Storage

1. Explain how to prepare a basic food plan and list food shopping guidelines

Make a basic food plan for Monday through Friday. Include breakfast, lunch, dinner, and snacks.

MONDAY

Breakfast

Snack

Lunch

Snack

Dinner

Snack

TUESDAY

Breakfast

Snack

Lunch

Snack

Dinner

Snack

WEDNESDAY

Breakfast

Snack

Lunch

Snack

Dinner

Snack

THURSDAY

Breakfast

Snack

Lunch

Snack

Dinner

Snack

FRIDAY

Breakfast

Snack

Lunch

Snack

Dinner

Snack

Name: _____

Fill in the Blank.

1. Avoid _____ or ready-made foods because they are more expensive.

2. If you have the time, make food from scratch and buy _____ items.

3. Read _____ for ingredients that may be harmful to your client.

4. Estimate the _____ by dividing the total cost by the number of servings.

5. For clients on a low-fat diet, take the _____ off chicken and turkey parts.

6. Buy fresh foods that are in season when they are at their _____ flavor.

7. Large amounts or larger sizes are usually more _____.

8. Cheaper cuts of meat tend to have more _____ in bones and fat.

Short Answer.

9. List four factors to consider when buying food.

_____
_____
_____
_____

2. List guidelines for safe food preparation

True or False.

Mark each statement with either a "T" for true or an "F" for false.

1. _____ You should wash your hands before, but not after, handling food.

2. _____ Sponges can be washed in the dishwasher to disinfect them.

3. _____ Defrost frozen foods on the countertops.

4. _____ Food can be left out safely for five hours.

5. _____ You need to cook poultry thoroughly to kill microorganisms.

6. _____ Food-borne illnesses affect up to one million people each year.

7. _____ It is best to use plastic cutting boards for raw meat.

8. _____ It is not necessary to change knives between cutting fresh meat and vegetables.

9. _____ It is especially important to prepare food safely for people who have weakened immune systems.

10. _____ Elderly people are at increased risk for a food-borne illness because often they can't taste if food is spoiled.

3. Identify methods of food preparation

Fill in the Blank.

Read the following descriptions and identify what method of food preparation it is. The methods are listed below. Some methods will be used more than once.

baking	microwaving
boiling	poaching
broiling	roasting
frying	sauteing
steaming	

1. _____ Safe for defrosting, reheating, and cooking, but this method can cause "cold spots."

2. _____ Cooked in barely boiling water or other liquids, this is an ideal way to prepare fish and eggs.

3. _____ Used mostly for meats and poultry, this method requires basting.

4. _____ This is a healthy way to prepare vegetables.

5. _____ Used mostly for meats, it involves cooking food close to the source of heat at a high temperature for a short time.

6. _____ The best method for cooking pasta, noodles, and rice.

7. _____ Done in a moderate oven, this method is used for many foods such as breads, fish, and vegetables.

8. _____ A quick way to cook vegetables and meats by using a small amount of oil in a frying pan and stirring constantly.

9. _____ A small amount of water is boiled in the bottom of a saucepan and food is set over it on a rack.

10. _____ The least healthy way to cook, this method uses a lot of fat.

11. _____ You can use this method to melt cheese or brown the top of a casserole.

4. Identify four methods of low-fat food preparation

Fill in the Blank.

1. _____ allows fats in meat to drip out before food is consumed, which lowers fat content.

2. Plan meals around _____, which are the base of the food pyramid.

3. Sometimes high-fat ingredients can be _____ to lower the fat content of a recipe.

4. _____ meat on paper towels after you brown it.

5. Leave out _____ on sandwiches or on top of casseroles.

6. An example of a low-fat meal based on grains is beans and _____.

7. Boiling, steaming, broiling, and _____ are all methods of cooking that require little fat.

8. Try substituting _____ for mayonnaise or sour cream.

5. List four guidelines for safe food storage

Multiple Choice.

Circle the letter of the answer that best completes the statement or answers the question.

1. After shopping, which foods should be put away first?
   a. meats
   b. dairy
   c. grains
   d. both a and b
   e. none of the above

2. It is a good idea to keep easily-spoiled items in the:
   a. door of the refrigerator
   b. cupboard
   c. rear of the refrigerator
   d. pantry
   e. none of the above

3. Refrigerator temperature should be at:
   a. 0 F
   b. 36°F - 40°F
   c. 10°F - 20°F
   d. either a or b
   e. none of the above

4. You can safely leave foods out for _____ hours.
   a. five
   b. three
   c. two
   d. twelve
   e. none of the above

5. If you are not sure whether food is spoiled, you should:
   a. discard it
   b. serve it and see if anyone complains or feels ill
   c. cook it for a longer time than usual
   d. all of the above
   e. none of the above

6. Describe guidelines for assisting with eating

Multiple Choice.

Circle the correct response.

1. When assisting clients with eating, encourage them to do whatever they can for themselves. This includes:
   a. if a client can hold a napkin, she should
   b. if a client can use special adaptive utensils, she should
   c. if a client can hold and eat finger foods, she should
   d. all of the above

2. Ways to promote a client's dignity while feeding include:
   a. Telling him, "Hurry up. I've still got to give you a bath."
   b. Asking him, "What would you like to try first?"
   c. Looking around the room while he is eating
   d. none of the above

True or False.

Mark each statement with either a "T" for true or an "F" for false.

3. _____ Clients who must be fed are often embarrassed and depressed about their dependence on another person.

4. _____ Alternate food and drink while feeding.

5. _____ Sit higher than a client while feeding.

6. _____ You should give a client your full attention during eating.

7. _____ When feeding a client, make sure the client's mouth is empty before giving another bite of food or sip of beverage.

8. _____ A client should be fed lying flat on his back.

Short Answer.

9. In a few words, describe how you might feel if you needed help to perform activities of daily living (ADLs), such as eating or bathing.

_____
_____
_____
_____
_____
_____
_____
_____
_____
_____
_____

7. Describe eating and swallowing problems a client may have

Short Answer.

1. List five ways to prevent aspiration.

   _____
   _____
   _____
   _____
   _____
   _____
   _____
   _____
   _____
   _____
   _____
   _____
   _____

Fill in the Blank.

2. A _____ tube is inserted into the nose going to the stomach. A _____ tube is inserted through the abdomen, into the stomach. With _____ a client receives nutrients directly into the bloodstream.

Name: _____

24

Managing Time, Energy, and Money

1. Explain three ways to work more efficiently

Short Answer.

1. For each of the three ways of working more efficiently described in this learning objective, give an example (other than what it is in the book) of how you can put the method into action.

2. List five ways to conserve time and energy.

2. Describe how to follow an established work plan with the client and family

Pick the busiest day you will have next week, and draft a work plan for that day. List tasks to complete and prioritize them.

3. Discuss ways to handle inappropriate requests

Scenario.

Read the following scenario and answer the question.

Richard, a home health aide, is preparing to leave his client's home for the day. Mr. Perez, his client, demands that Richard buy him some soup at the grocery store before he leaves. This errand is not in the care plan, but Mr. Perez tells him that he really wants some soup. Mr. Perez begins to cry. What should Richard do in this situation?

Name: _____

4. List five money-saving homemaking tips

Short Answer.

List and briefly explain the five money-saving tips.

_____
_____
_____
_____
_____
_____
_____
_____
_____
_____
_____
_____

5. List guidelines for handling a client's money

Short Answer.

1. What are your state's guidelines for handling a client's money?

_____
_____
_____
_____

True or False.

Mark each statement with either a "T" for true or an "F" for false.

2. _____ It is fine to use your client's money for your own things as long as you pay it back.

3. _____ Use cash whenever possible.

4. _____ It is a good idea to estimate the amount of money you will need before you request it.

5. _____ Return receipts to client or family member as soon as possible.

6. _____ It is a good idea to keep a record of the money you've spent and where you've spent it.

7. _____ You are not responsible for lost money.

8. _____ Keep a client's cash separate from yours.

9. _____ If a client is unsure about their budget, you should give them advice about how much to spend and where to spend it.

Name: _____

25

Caring for Yourself and Your Career

1. Explain how to conduct a job search

Short Answer.

List three resources you should try when looking for potential employers.

_____

_____

_____

2. Identify documents that may be required when applying for a job

Short Answer.

List four documents that you may need when you apply for a job.

_____

_____

_____

_____

3. Demonstrate completing an effective job application

Complete the sample job application.

Employment Application

Personal Information

Name:	Date:
Social Security Number:	
Home Address:	
City, state, Zip:	
Home Phone:	Business Phone:
US Citizen?	If Not Give Visa No. & expiration:

Position Applying For

Title	Salary Desired:
Referred By:	Date Available:

Education

High School (Name, City, State):	
Graduation Date:	
Technical or Undergraduate School:	
Dates Attended:	Degree Major:

References

4. Demonstrate competence in job interview techniques

Write "Yes" or "No" next to the descriptions below to indicate whether or not it is appropriate for a job interview.

1. _____ Arrives a couple of minutes late for the interview.
2. _____ Looks happy to be there.
3. _____ Asks, "Do you mind if I smoke?"
4. _____ Wears very little jewelry
5. _____ Asks, "How many hours would I work?"
6. _____ Brings child with her since she could not find a babysitter
7. _____ Says, "I won't work with patients with AIDS."
8. _____ Sits up straight
9. _____ Asks, "What benefits do I receive with this job?"
10. _____ Shakes hands with interviewer
11. _____ Eats a granola bar during the interview
12. _____ Asks, "Did I get the job?

5. Discuss appropriate responses to criticism

Read the following and mark whether they are examples of hostile or constructive criticism. Use an "H" for hostile and a "C" for constructive.

1. _____ "You are a horrible person."
2. _____ "If you weren't so slow, things might get done around here."
3. _____ "Some of your reports are not completed; try to be more accurate."
4. _____ "That was the worst meal I've ever eaten!"
5. _____ "I don't think you caught my meaning. Let me put it differently."
6. _____ "Where did you learn how to clean?"
7. _____ "That was a stupid idea."
8. _____ "That procedure could have been performed in a more efficient way."
9. _____ "Try to make more of an effort to listen."
10. _____ "Stop being so lazy."

6. Identify effective ways to make a complaint to an employer or supervisor

Scenario.

Read the following scenario and answer the question.

Anne is a home health aide who works three days a week for her client, Mrs. Singer. Generally, Mrs. Singer's son, Wayne, is there as well, and he and Anne work as a team. Wayne finds a new job and cannot be home during the day anymore. The next time Anne arrives, Mrs. Singer is moody and distant. She is reluctant to follow the care plan and she tells Anne that she will not take a bath until Wayne comes home. She also refuses to eat food that Anne has cooked, insisting she can only eat her son's cooking. After some gentle urging, Anne gets Mrs. Singer to eat and take a bath.

The next time Anne works, Mrs. Singer drops her plate on the floor and tells Anne that she is a lousy cook. She tells her to fix a new meal and clean up the mess. Anne does both, although she feels very upset.

Should this be reported to a supervisor? If so, how?

_____

_____

_____

_____

_____

_____

_____

Name: _____

7. Identify guidelines for making job changes

Fill in the Blank.

1. You should always give your employer _____ weeks written notice that you will be leaving.

2. Potential future employers may talk with your past _____.

3. If you decide to change jobs, be _____.

8. List your state's requirements for maintaining certification

Short Answer.

1. How many hours of in-service education are required each year by your state?

2. How long is an absence from working allowed, without retraining, by your state?

9. Describe continuing education for home health aides

True or False.

Mark each statement with either a "T" for true or an "F" for false.

1. _____ The federal government requires 20 hours of continuing education each year.

2. _____ Treatments or regulations can change.

3. _____ States require less continuing education than the federal government.

4. _____ In-service continuing education courses help you keep your knowledge fresh.

Short Answer.

5. List three of the responsibilities a home health aide has for receiving continuing education.

10. Define stress and stressors, and list examples

Short Answer.

What are some things that make you experience stress? How do you react when you're stressed?

11. Explain ways to manage stress

Multiple Choice.

Circle the letter of the answer that best completes the statement or answers the question.

1. Stress is a(n) _____ response.
   a. relaxation
   b. emotional
   c. physical
   d. both b and c
   e. all of the above

2. When your heart beats fast in stressful situations, it can be a result of the increase of the hormone
   a. testosterone
   b. estrogen
   c. adrenaline
   d. progesterone
   e. none of the above

3. Which of the following is NOT a physical result of the effects of stress?
   a. increase in heart rate
   b. increase in blood pressure
   c. increase in respiratory rate
   d. increase in nervous system response
   e. none of the above

4. A healthy lifestyle is the result of:
   a. eating when you're not hungry
   b. exercising regularly
   c. smoking a few cigarettes a week
   d. all of the above
   e. none of the above

5. Which of the following is a sign that you are not managing stress?
   a. abusing a client
   b. not being able to focus on your work
   c. not getting along with your co-workers
   d. all of the above
   e. none of the above

Short Answer.

6. List four places and/or people to whom you can turn to help you manage stress.
   _____
   _____
   _____
   _____

12. Demonstrate two effective relaxation techniques

Fill in the Blank.

1. When doing the body scan exercise, pay attention to breathing and _____.

2. A _____ exercise can help you feel refreshed in a short time.

3. When performing the waterfall exercise, breathe deeply and imagine the force of the water is washing away your _____.

4. Start at the balls of your _____ when doing the body scan relaxation exercise.

13. Describe how to develop a personal stress management plan

Short Answer.

Write out your own personal stress management plan. Be sure to include things like diet, exercise, relaxation exercise, entertainment, etc.

_____
_____
_____
_____
_____
_____
_____
_____
_____

Name: _____

121

_____ debt is often the highest interest charged on any loan.

2. _____ some amount every time you get a check. Ten percent is a good goal.

3. Reduce or avoid _____, such as to banks, mortgage companies, or credit card companies.

5. Set a cash _____ for the week and stick to it.

14. List five guidelines for managing time

Short Answer.

List five guidelines for managing time.

_____
_____
_____
_____
_____

15. Demonstrate an understanding of the basics of money management

Crossword.

Across

1. When you apply for a mortgage or car loan, the bank or lender will check your _____.

2. To control expenses, try writing down what you _____ each day.

4. Very few people _____ their money well.

6. Making a personal or household _____ helps you start solving money problems.

Down

1. The interest charged on _____

16. Demonstrate an understanding that money matters are emotional

Short Answer.

When was the last time you wanted something you could not afford? How did it make you feel? What did you do?

_____
_____
_____
_____
_____
_____
_____

Name: _____

17. List ways to remind yourself that your work is important, valuable, and meaningful

Short Answer.

What made you choose to be a home health aide?

Name: _____

PROCEDURE CHECKLISTS

5

Infection Control and Standard Precautions

Putting on gloves

✓ **Procedure Steps**

- [ ] 1. Washes hands.
- [ ] 2. If right-handed, slides one glove on left hand (reverse, if left-handed).
- [ ] 3. With gloved hand takes second glove and slides other hand into the glove.
- [ ] 4. Interlaces fingers to smooth out folds and create a comfortable fit.
- [ ] 5. Carefully looks for tears, holes, or spots. Replaces the glove if necessary.
- [ ] 6. If wearing a gown, pulls the cuff of the gloves over the sleeve of gown.

Comments:

Taking off gloves

✓ **Procedure Steps**

- [ ] 1. Touches only the outside of one glove and pulls the first glove off, turning it inside out.
- [ ] 2. With ungloved hand, reaches two fingers inside the remaining glove. Does not touch any part of the outside.
- [ ] 3. Pulls down, turning this glove inside out and over the first glove.
- [ ] 4. Disposes of gloves properly.
- [ ] 5. Washes hands.

Comments:

Putting on a gown

✓ **Procedure Steps**

- [ ] 1. Washes hands.
- [ ] 2. Opens gown without shaking it. Slips arms into the sleeves and pulls gown on.
- [ ] 3. Ties neck ties.
- [ ] 4. Pulls gown until it completely covers clothing. Ties the back ties.

Comments:

Putting on mask and eye shield

✓ **Procedure Steps**

- [ ] 1. Washes hands.
- [ ] 2. Picks up mask by top strings or elastic strap. Does not touch mask where it touches face.
- [ ] 3. Adjusts mask over nose and mouth. Ties top strings first, then bottom strings.
- [ ] 4. Puts on eye shield.

Comments:

Disinfecting using wet heat

✓ **Procedure Steps**

- [ ] 1. Washes hands.

Name: _____

- ☐ 2. Places items in the pot and fills it with water, covering all items.
- ☐ 3. Places lid on pot and places pot on stove.
- ☐ 4. Turns on heat and brings water to a boil. Boils for 20 minutes.
- ☐ 5. Turns off heat. Allows items and water to cool.
- ☐ 6. After items have cooled, removes cover and then items. Places items on rack or towel to dry.
- ☐ 7. Washes and dries equipment. Returns to proper storage.
- ☐ 8. Washes hands.
- ☐ 9. Documents procedure.

Comments:

Disinfecting using dry heat

✓ **Procedure Steps**

- ☐ 1. Washes hands.
- ☐ 2. Places items in the pan and places pan or sheet in oven.
- ☐ 3. Turns on oven to 350° F and bakes for one hour.
- ☐ 4. Turns off heat. Allow items to cool.
- ☐ 5. After items have cooled, removes items.
- ☐ 6. Stores items.
- ☐ 7. Washes and dries equipment. Returns to proper storage.
- ☐ 8. Washes hands.
- ☐ 9. Documents procedure.

Comments:

7

Emergency Care and Disaster Preparation

Heimlich maneuver for the conscious person

✓ **Procedure Steps**

- ☐ 1. Stands behind person and brings arms under person's arms. Wraps arms around person's waist.
- ☐ 2. Makes a fist with one hand. Places flat, thumb side of the fist against person's abdomen, above the navel but below the breastbone.
- ☐ 3. Grasps the fist with other hand. Pulls both hands toward self and up, quickly and forcefully.
- ☐ 4. Repeats until object is pushed out or person loses consciousness.
- ☐ 5. Reports and documents incident.

Comments:

Clearing an obstructed airway in a conscious infant

✓ **Procedure Steps**

- ☐ 1. Lies the infant face down on forearm; if sitting, rests the arm holding the infant's torso on lap or thigh. Supports infant's jaw and head with your hand.
- ☐ 2. Delivers up to 5 back blows.
- ☐ 3. If the obstruction is not expelled, turns infant onto his back while supporting the head. Delivers up to 5 chest thrusts
- ☐ 4. Repeats, alternating 5 back blows and 5 chest compressions until object is pushed out or the infant loses consciousness.

Name: _____   125

❏ 5. Reports and documents incident.

Comments:

Shock

✓ **Procedure Steps**

❏ 1. Has the person lie down on her back unless bleeding from the mouth or vomiting.

❏ 2. Controls bleeding if bleeding occurs.

❏ 3. Checks pulse and respirations if possible.

❏ 4. Keeps person as calm and comfortable as possible.

❏ 5. Maintains normal body temperature.

❏ 6. Elevates the feet unless person has a head or abdominal injury, breathing difficulties, or a fractured bone or back.

❏ 7. Does not give person anything to eat or drink.

❏ 8. Calls for help immediately.

❏ 9. Reports and documents incident.

Comments:

Heart attack

✓ **Procedure Steps**

❏ 1. Calls or has someone call emergency services. Calls supervisor.

❏ 2. Places person in a comfortable position. Encourages him to rest, and reassures him that he will not be left alone.

❏ 3. Loosens clothing around the neck.

❏ 4. Does not give person liquids.

❏ 5. If person takes heart medication, such as nitroglycerin, finds medication and offers it to him. Does not place medication in person's mouth.

❏ 6. Monitors person's breathing and pulse. If breathing stops or person has no pulse, performs rescue breathing or CPR if trained to do so.

❏ 7. Stays with person until help arrives.

❏ 8. Reports and documents incident.

Comments:

Bleeding

✓ **Procedure Steps**

❏ 1. Puts on gloves.

❏ 2. Holds thick sterile pad or a clean cloth against the wound.

❏ 3. Presses down hard directly on the bleeding wound until help arrives. Does not decrease pressure. Puts additional pads over the first pad if blood seeps through. Does not remove the first pad.

❏ 4. Raises the wound above the heart to slow down the bleeding.

❏ 5. When bleeding is under control, secures the dressing to keep it in place. Checks person for symptoms of shock. Stays with person until help arrives.

❏ 6. Washes hands.

❏ 7. Reports and documents incident.

Comments:

Poisoning

✓ **Procedure Steps**

❏ 1. Looks for a container that will help determine what the client has taken or eaten. Checks the mouth for chemical burns and notes breath odor.

Name: _____

- ❏ 2. Calls the local or state poison control center immediately. Follows instructions.
- ❏ 3. Notifies supervisor.
- ❏ 4. Reports and documents incident.

Comments:

Burns

✓ **Procedure Steps**

Minor burns:

- ❏ 1. Uses cool, clean water (not ice) to decrease the skin temperature and prevent further injury (does not use ointment, salve, or grease).
- ❏ 2. Dampens a clean cloth and covers burn.
- ❏ 3. Covers area with a dry, sterile gauze.

Serious burns:

- ❏ 1. Removes person from the source of burn.
- ❏ 2. Checks for breathing, pulse, and severe bleeding.
- ❏ 3. Calls for emergency help.
- ❏ 4. Removes as much clothing around the burn as possible and covers burn with thick, dry, sterile gauze or a clean cloth (does not apply water or use ointment, salve, or grease).
- ❏ 5. Elevates affected part after person lies down.
- ❏ 6. If the burn is covers a larger area, wraps person in a dry, clean sheet and applies ice pack. Takes care not to rub the skin.
- ❏ 7. Waits for emergency medical help.
- ❏ 8. Reports and documents incident.

Comments:

Seizures

✓ **Procedure Steps**

- ❏ 1. Lowers person to the floor.
- ❏ 2. Has someone call emergency services immediately. Does not leave person unless has to get medical help.
- ❏ 3. Moves furniture away to prevent injury. If a pillow is nearby, places it under his head.
- ❏ 4. Does not try to restrain the person.
- ❏ 5. Does not force anything between the person's teeth. Does not place hands in person's mouth.
- ❏ 6. Does not give liquids.
- ❏ 7. When the seizure is over, checks breathing.
- ❏ 8. Reports and documents incident.

Comments:

Fainting

✓ **Procedure Steps**

- ❏ 1. Has person lie down or sit down before fainting occurs.
- ❏ 2. If person is in sitting position, has him bend forward and place his head between his knees. If person is lying flat on his back, elevates the legs.
- ❏ 3. Loosens any tight clothing.
- ❏ 4. Has person stay in position for at least five minutes after symptoms disappear.
- ❏ 5. Helps person get up slowly. Continues to observe him for symptoms of fainting.
- ❏ 6. Reports and documents incident.

Comments:

Name: _____

127

Nosebleed

✓ **Procedure Steps**

☐ 1. Elevates head of the bed or tells client to remain in sitting position. Offers tissues or a clean cloth.

☐ 2. Puts on gloves. Applies firm pressure over the bridge of the nose. Squeezes bridge of nose with thumb and forefinger.

☐ 3. Applies pressure consistently until bleeding stops.

☐ 4. Uses a cool cloth or ice wrapped in a cloth on back of neck, forehead, or upper lip to slow blood flow.

☐ 5. Reports and documents incident.

Comments:

Helping a client who has fallen

✓ **Procedure Steps**

☐ 1. Assesses client's condition and gets help if condition warrants it.

☐ 2. Looks for broken bones.

☐ 3. Asks client to move each body part separately to observe.

☐ 4. Makes client comfortable.

☐ 5. Calls supervisor and report accurately.

Comments:

12

Transfers, Ambulation, and Positioning

Assisting a client to a dangling position

✓ **Procedure Steps**

☐ 1. Washes hands.

☐ 2. Explains procedure to client.

☐ 3. Provides privacy.

☐ 4. Adjusts the bed to a comfortable working height, if possible. Locks bed wheels.

☐ 5. Folds back top covers. Asks client to roll on side.

☐ 6. Assists client to dangling position, providing help as necessary. Observes client for dizziness.

☐ 7. Assists client to put on nonskid shoes.

☐ 8. Returns client safely to bed or completes transfer.

☐ 9. Returns bed to lowest position if raised.

☐ 10. Washes hands.

☐ 11. Documents procedure and any observations.

Comments:

Helping a client sit up using the arm lock

✓ **Procedure Steps**

☐ 1. Washes hands.

☐ 2. Explains procedure to client.

☐ 3. Provides privacy.

☐ 4. Adjusts the bed to a comfortable working height, if possible. Locks bed wheels.

☐ 5. Stands facing the bed with feet apart and knees bent.

☐ 6. Grasps client in the arm lock position.

☐ 7. Reaches under client's head and places other hand on client's far shoulder. Has client bend knees. Bends own knees.

Name: _____

☐ 8. Rocks backward at the count of three and pulls client to sitting position.

☐ 9. Observes client for dizziness.

☐ 10. Returns bed to lowest position if raised.

☐ 11. Washes hands.

☐ 12. Documents procedure and any observations.

Comments:

Helping a client stand up

✓ **Procedure Steps**

☐ 1. Washes hands.

☐ 2. Explains procedure to client.

☐ 3. Provides privacy.

☐ 4. Adjusts the bed to a comfortable working height, if possible. Locks bed wheels.

☐ 5. Assists client to dangling position.

☐ 6. Puts nonskid footwear on client.

☐ 7. If client requires little or no assistance, steadies client as he or she pushes up to the standing position.

☐ 8. If client requires assistance, places one foot between client's feet with knees bent, and places arms around client's waist, with client leaning forward.

☐ 9. Rocks weight onto back foot on count of three and assists client to stand up.

☐ 10. Observes client for dizziness.

☐ 11. Washes hands.

☐ 12. Documents procedure and any observations.

Comments:

Using a transfer belt to assist with ambulation

✓ **Procedure Steps**

☐ 1. Washes hands.

☐ 2. Explains procedure to client.

☐ 3. Provides privacy.

☐ 4. Adjusts the bed to a comfortable working height, if possible. Locks bed wheels.

☐ 5. Places transfer belt around client's waist over clothing.

☐ 6. Puts nonskid footwear on client.

☐ 7. Assists client to standing position.

☐ 8. Stands behind and to the side of client, holding onto the belt. Offers support as necessary.

☐ 9. Observes the client for dizziness or fatigue.

☐ 10. Returns the client safely to bed or a chair and positions client comfortably.

☐ 11. Washes hands.

☐ 12. Documents procedure and any observations.

Comments:

Assisting with ambulation for a client who uses a cane or walker

✓ **Procedure Steps**

☐ 1. Washes hands.

☐ 2. Explains procedure to client.

☐ 3. Provides privacy.

☐ 4. Adjusts the bed to a comfortable working height, if possible. Locks bed wheels.

☐ 5. Fastens transfer belt around the client's waist over clothing.

☐ 6. Puts nonskid footwear on client.

Name: _____

- ☐ 7. Assists client to standing position.
- ☐ 8. Assists client with ambulation as necessary, walking slightly behind or on the weak side of client.
- ☐ 9. Watches for obstacles in the client's path.
- ☐ 10. Lets the client set the pace, encouraging rest as necessary.
- ☐ 11. Returns the client safely to bed or a chair and positions client comfortably.
- ☐ 12. Washes hands.
- ☐ 13. Documents procedure and any observations.

Comments:

Helping a client move from a bed to a chair

✓ **Procedure Steps**

- ☐ 1. Washes hands.
- ☐ 2. Explains procedure to client.
- ☐ 3. Provides privacy.
- ☐ 4. Assists client to dangle.
- ☐ 5. Positions chair on client's stronger side at an angle. If using wheelchair, locks brakes and removes foot rests.
- ☐ 6. Assists client to standing position.
- ☐ 7. Instructs client to take small steps to the chair while turning around and then grasping one arm of the chair. Assists client to pivot if necessary.
- ☐ 8. Assists client to lower himself into the chair.
- ☐ 9. Positions client comfortably, checking for good alignment and placing robe or blanket over lap. For wheelchairs, replaces foot rests and places client's feet on them.
- ☐ 10. Washes hands.

- ☐ 11. Documents procedure and any observations.

Comments:

Helping a client transfer using a slide board

✓ **Procedure Steps**

- ☐ 1. Washes hands.
- ☐ 2. Explains procedure to client.
- ☐ 3. Provides privacy.
- ☐ 4. Assists client to dangle.
- ☐ 5. Positions chair on client's stronger side at an angle. If using wheelchair, locks brakes and removes foot rests.
- ☐ 6. Instructs client to lean away from the transfer side.
- ☐ 7. Places one end of slide board under client's buttocks and thigh and the other end on the surface to which client is transferring.
- ☐ 8. Instructs client to push up with hands and scoot across the board.
- ☐ 9. If client needs assistance, braces client's knees, grasps the transfer belt, and instructs client to lean forward. Assists client to scoot across the board, without dragging client.
- ☐ 10. Removes sliding board after transfer is complete. Positions client comfortably, checking for good alignment.
- ☐ 11. Washes hands.
- ☐ 12. Documents procedure and any observations.

Comments:

Name: _____

Transferring a client using a mechanical lift

✓ **Procedure Steps**

☐ 1. Washes hands.

☐ 2. Explains procedure to client.

☐ 3. Provides privacy.

☐ 4. Positions wheelchair next to bed and locks brakes.

☐ 5. Positions sling under client, rolling client to one side of bed and then the other.

☐ 6. Positions mechanical lift next to bed, opening the base to its widest point and pushing of lift under bed. Positions overhead bar directly over client.

☐ 7. Attaches straps to sling properly.

☐ 8. Raises client in sling two inches above bed, following manufacturer's instructions. Allows client to gain equilibrium.

☐ 9. Rolls mechanical lift to position client over chair or wheelchair. Lifting partner supports and guides client's body.

☐ 10. Slowly lowers client into chair or wheelchair, pushing down gently on client's knees.

☐ 11. Undoes straps from overhead bar to sling, leaving sling in place.

☐ 12. Positions client comfortably, checking for good alignment.

☐ 13. Washes hands.

☐ 14. Documents procedure and any observations.

Comments:

Turning a client in bed

✓ **Procedure Steps**

☐ 1. Washes hands.

☐ 2. Explains procedure to client.

☐ 3. Provides privacy.

☐ 4. Adjusts the bed to a comfortable working height, if possible. Locks bed wheels.

☐ 5. Makes sure client is in supine position and centered in the bed. Stands at the side of the bed client will face. Places client's hand palm up under the hip.

☐ 6. Lifts client's far leg over the near leg, flexing the knee.

☐ 7. Assumes a good stance.

☐ 8. Grasps client's far shoulder and far hip. Counts to three, rocking weight forward and back, and rolls client onto side.

☐ 9. Positions client comfortably using pillows or other supports, and checks for good alignment.

☐ 10. Washes hands.

☐ 11. Documents procedure and any observations.

Comments:

Moving a client up in bed

✓ **Procedure Steps**

If client can assist:

☐ 1. Washes hands.

☐ 2. Explains procedure to client.

☐ 3. Provides privacy.

☐ 4. Adjusts the bed to comfortable working height, if possible. Lowers head of bed. Locks bed wheels. Raises side rail on far side of bed. Removes the pillow for later use.

☐ 5. Places one arm under client's shoulders and the other under client's buttocks.

☐ 6. Instructs client to bend knees and push down with his feet on the count of three.

☐ 7. Assists client to move toward the head of the bed on the count of three.

Name: _____

- [ ] 8. Positions client comfortably, arranges pillow and blankets, and returns bed to lowest position.
- [ ] 9. Washes hands.
- [ ] 10. Documents procedure and any observations.

Comments:

If client cannot assist:

- [ ] 1. Washes hands.
- [ ] 2. Explains procedure to client.
- [ ] 3. Provides privacy.
- [ ] 4. Adjusts the bed to comfortable working height, if possible. Lowers head of bed. Locks bed wheels. Raises both side rails.
- [ ] 5. Stands behind the bed with feet apart and one foot slightly in front of other.
- [ ] 6. Rolls and grasps top of draw sheet, bends knees, keeping back straight, and rocks weight from front foot to back foot.
- [ ] 7. Positions client comfortably, arranges pillow and blankets, unrolls draw sheet, and returns bed to lowest position.
- [ ] 8. Washes hands.
- [ ] 9. Documents procedure and any observations.

Comments:

When you have help from another person and client cannot assist:

- [ ] 1. Washes hands.
- [ ] 2. Explains procedure to client.
- [ ] 3. Provides privacy.
- [ ] 4. Adjusts the bed to comfortable working height, if possible. Lowers head of bed. Locks bed wheels.
- [ ] 5. Stands behind the bed with feet apart and one foot slightly in front of other.
- [ ] 6. Rolls and grasps top of draw sheet, bends knees, keeping back straight, and rocks weight from front foot to back foot.
- [ ] 7. Positions client comfortably, arranges pillow and blankets, unrolls draw sheet, and returns bed to lowest position.
- [ ] 8. Washes hands.
- [ ] 9. Documents procedure and any observations.

Comments:

Logrolling a client

✓ **Procedure Steps**

- [ ] 1. Washes hands.
- [ ] 2. Explains procedure to client.
- [ ] 3. Provides privacy.
- [ ] 4. Adjusts the bed to comfortable working height, if possible. Lowers head of bed. Locks bed wheels.
- [ ] 5. Moves client to one side of the bed by moving the head and shoulders, then the hips and legs towards self.
- [ ] 6. Makes sure client's body is in good alignment.
- [ ] 7. If available, raises side rail on the side of the bed client is now closest to.
- [ ] 8. Moves to the other side of the bed and lowers side rail if available. Assumes a good stance.
- [ ] 9. With knees bent, grasps client with one hand on far hip and one on far shoulder. Rolls the client onto side.
- [ ] 10. Positions client comfortably with pillows or supports, and checks for good align-

ment. Raises side rail. Returns bed to lowest position.

☐ 11. Washes hands.

☐ 12. Documents procedure and any observations.

Comments:

Giving a back rub

✓ **Procedure Steps**

☐ 1. Washes hands.

☐ 2. Explains procedure to client.

☐ 3. Provides privacy.

☐ 4. Adjusts the bed to comfortable working height, if possible. Lowers head of bed. Locks bed wheels.

☐ 5. Instructs client to lie in prone position or side position. Covers client with blanket and folds back bed covers, exposing client's back to the top of the buttocks. If client is lying on side, places towel along the length of his back.

☐ 6. Warms lotion and hands, and warns client that lotion may still feel cool.

☐ 7. Pours lotion onto hands and rubs hands together.

☐ 8. Starting at the upper part of the buttocks, makes long, smooth upward strokes with both hands. Circles hands up along spine, shoulders, and then back down along the outer edges of the back.

☐ 9. Repeats for three to five minutes.

☐ 10. Starting at the base of the spine, makes kneading motions using the first two fingers and thumb of each hand. Circles hands up along spine, circling at shoulders and buttocks.

☐ 11. Gently massages bony areas. Massages around any red areas, rather than on them.

Name: _____

☐ 12. Lets client know when back rub is almost completed.

☐ 13. Dries the back and applies powder, if appropriate.

☐ 14. Removes blanket and towel, assists client with getting dressed, and positions client comfortably. Returns bed to lowest position.

☐ 15. Stores lotion and disposes of dirty linens properly.

☐ 16. Washes hands.

☐ 17. Documents procedure and any observations.

Comments:

13

Personal Care Skills

Helping the client transfer to the bathtub

✓ **Procedure Steps**

☐ 1. Washes hands.

☐ 2. Explains procedure to client.

☐ 3. Helps client to the bathroom.

☐ 4. Provides privacy.

☐ 5. Seats client in chair facing tub. If using wheelchair, locks brakes and raises foot rests.

☐ 6. Places client's legs over sides of tub.

☐ 7. Brings client to sitting position on edge of tub properly.

☐ 8. Lowers client into tub properly, assisting as necessary.

☐ 9. Reverses procedure to help client out of tub.

Name: _____

10. Washes hands.

11. Documents procedure and any observations.

Comments:

Helping the ambulatory client take a shower or tub bath

✓ **Procedure Steps**

1. Washes hands.
2. Explains procedure to client.
3. Cleans tub if necessary, places mat, and sets up tub or shower chair. Places non-skid rug next to tub.
4. Provides privacy.
5. Puts on gloves if client has broken skin.
6. Fills tub with warm water (105°F to 110°F on bath thermometer) or adjusts shower water temperature.
7. Assists client to undress as necessary and helps client to tub or shower.
8. If client is able to bathe alone, places supplies and signal near client. Checks on client every five minutes.
9. If showering, stays with client and assists.
10. Assists client as necessary, washing from clean to dirty areas. Assists with rinsing.
11. Assists with shampooing.
12. Helps client out and assists client with drying if necessary.
13. Helps client to bed.
14. Cleans tub.
15. Washes hands.
16. Puts supplies away.
17. Documents procedure and any observations.

Comments:

Assisting with a bed bath

✓ **Procedure Steps**

1. Washes hands.
2. Explains procedure to client.
3. Provides privacy.
4. Adjusts the bed to a comfortable working height, if possible. Locks bed wheels.
5. Asks client to remove glasses and jewelry. Offers bedpan.
6. Places blanket over client and checks sheets.
7. Fills basin and checks temperature (105°F to 110°F).
8. Puts on gloves if client has open lesions or wounds.
9. Asks and assists client to participate in washing.
10. Uncovers only one part of the body at a time. Places a towel under the body part being washed.
11. Washes, rinses, and dries one part of the body at a time. Starts at the head, working down, and completing front first.

Eyes and Face:

☐ Washes face with wet washcloth (no soap) beginning with the eyes, using a different area of the washcloth for each eye, washing inner aspect to outer aspect. Washes the face from the middle outward using firm but gentle strokes. Washes neck and ears and behind the ears. Rinses and pats dry.

Arms:

☐ Washes arm and underarm. Uses long strokes from the shoulder down to the elbow. Rinses and pats dry. Washes the elbow. Washes, rinses, and dries from the elbow down to the wrist.

- [ ] Washes hand in a basin. Provides nail care if it has been assigned. Applies lotion if ordered.

Chest:

- [ ] Lifts the towel only enough to wash the chest, rinse it, and pat dry. For a female client: washes, rinses, and dries breasts and under breasts.

Abdomen:

- [ ] Washes abdomen, rinses and pats dry.

Legs:

- [ ] Washes the thigh. Uses long downward strokes. Rinses and pats dry. Does the same from the knee to the ankle.

- [ ] Washes the foot and between the toes in a basin. Rinses foot and pats dry. Provides nail care if it has been assigned. Applies lotion if ordered.

Back:

- [ ] Helps client move to the center of the bed, then turns onto his side so back is facing self. Washes back, neck, and buttocks with long, downward strokes. Rinses and pats dry. Applies lotion if ordered.

- [ ] 12. Puts on gloves before washing perineal area.

- [ ] 13. Changes bath water. Washes, rinses, and dries perineal area, working from front to back.

For a female client:

- [ ] Washes the perineum with soap and water from front to back, using single strokes. Uses a clean area of washcloth or clean washcloth for each stroke. Wipes the center of the perineum, then each side. Spreads the labia majora. Wipes from front to back on each side. Rinses the area in the same way. Dries entire perineal area moving from front to back, using a blotting motion with towel. Asks client to turn on her side. Washes, rinses, and dries buttocks and anal area. Cleanses anal area without contaminating the perineal area.

For a male client:

- [ ] If client is uncircumcised, retracts the foreskin first. Gently pushes skin towards the base of penis. Holds the penis by the shaft and washes in a circular motion from the tip down to the base. Uses a clean area of washcloth or clean washcloth for each stroke. Rinses the penis. Then washes the scrotum and groin. Rinses and pats dry. If client is uncircumcised, gently returns foreskin to normal position. Asks client to turn on his side. Washes, rinses, and dries buttocks and anal area. Cleanses anal area without contaminating the perineal area.

- [ ] 14. Disposes of water and gloves properly. Places soiled washcloths and towels in proper container.

- [ ] 15. Gives back rub if time permits.

- [ ] 16. Assist client with grooming as necessary. Returns bed to lowest position.

- [ ] 17. Washes and stores everything. Changes bed sheets and blankets.

- [ ] 18. Washes hands.

- [ ] 19. Documents procedure and any observations.

Comments:

Providing fingernail care

✓ **Procedure Steps**

- [ ] 1. Washes hands.
- [ ] 2. Explains procedure to client.
- [ ] 3. Provides privacy.
- [ ] 4. Adjusts the bed to a comfortable working height, if possible. Locks bed wheels.
- [ ] 5. Puts on gloves if client has broken skin.

Name: _____

❑ 6. Removes nail polish if necessary.
❑ 7. Fills basin with warm water (105°F).
❑ 8. Soaks the client's nails for two to four minutes.
❑ 9. Removes hands from water. Washes hands with soapy washcloth. Rinses. Dries client's hands with a towel, including between fingers.
❑ 10. Gently pushes back the cuticles using the flat end of the orangewood stick or a towel.
❑ 11. Cleans under nails with orangewood stick. Wipes orangewood stick on towel after each nail. Washes the hands again and dries.
❑ 12. Shapes fingernails with an emery board or nail file. Applies lotion.
❑ 13. Discards water and cleans basin. Disposes of towels in proper place and stores supplies. Returns bed to lowest position.
❑ 14. Washes hands.
❑ 15. Documents procedure and any observations.

Comments:

Providing foot care

✓ **Procedure Steps**

❑ 1. Washes hands.
❑ 2. Explains procedure to client.
❑ 3. Provides privacy.
❑ 4. Puts on gloves if client has broken skin.
❑ 5. Fills basin with warm water (105°F).
❑ 6. Soaks client's feet for ten minutes, adding warm water as necessary.
❑ 7. Removes one foot from water. Washes entire foot, including between the toes and around nail beds with soapy washcloth.
❑ 8. Rinses and dries entire foot, including between the toes, with a soapy washcloth. Applies lotion.
❑ 9. Repeats steps for other foot.
❑ 10. Observes condition of feet.
❑ 11. Assists client to replace socks.
❑ 12. Discards water and cleans basin. Disposes of towels properly.
❑ 13. Washes hands.
❑ 14. Documents procedure and any observations.

Comments:

Shampooing hair

✓ **Procedure Steps**

❑ 1. Washes hands.
❑ 2. Explains procedure to client.
❑ 3. Provides privacy.
❑ 4. Positions client in sink, tub, shower, or in bed, and wets hair.
❑ 5. Applies shampoo, and massages scalp.
❑ 6. Rinses hair. Repeats.
❑ 7. Wraps client's hair.
❑ 8. Removes towel and combs/brushes hair.
❑ 9. Dries and styles hair.
❑ 10. Washes and stores equipment. Removes gloves.
❑ 11. Washes hands.
❑ 12. Documents procedure and any observations.

Comments:

Name: _____

Helping a client shave

✓ **Procedure Steps**

- ❏ 1. Washes hands.
- ❏ 2. Explains procedure to client.
- ❏ 3. Provides privacy.
- ❏ 4. Puts on gloves.
- ❏ 5. Adjusts the bed to a comfortable working height, if possible. Locks bed wheels. Places equipment close by and places towel across chest.
- ❏ 6. If using an electric razor, turns on and shaves face, pulling skin tight.
- ❏ 7. If using a safety razor, softens beard, lathers face, and shaves in direction of hair growth.
- ❏ 8. Rinses face. Offers mirror. Applies aftershave if client desires.
- ❏ 9. Washes and stores equipment. Removes gloves. Returns bed to lowest position.
- ❏ 10. Washes hands.
- ❏ 11. Documents procedure and any observations.

Comments:

Combing or brushing hair

✓ **Procedure Steps**

- ❏ 1. Washes hands.
- ❏ 2. Explains procedure to client.
- ❏ 3. Provides privacy.
- ❏ 4. If confined to bed, raises head and places towel under it. Adjusts the bed to a comfortable working height, if possible. Locks bed wheels. If ambulatory, provides comfortable chair and places towel around shoulders.
- ❏ 5. Puts on gloves only if client has broken skin on the scalp or face.
- ❏ 6. If hair is tangled, detangles gently.
- ❏ 7. Brushes hair properly.
- ❏ 8. Styles hair in the way the client prefers. Offers a mirror to client.
- ❏ 9. Removes towel, and stores supplies. Removes gloves. Returns bed to lowest position.
- ❏ 10. Washes hands.
- ❏ 11. Documents procedure and any observations.

Comments:

Assisting with mouth care

✓ **Procedure Steps**

- ❏ 1. Washes hands.
- ❏ 2. Explains procedure to client.
- ❏ 3. Provides privacy.
- ❏ 4. If client is in bed, props him up. Adjusts the bed to a comfortable working height, if possible. Locks bed wheels. Places towel under head and across chest.
- ❏ 5. Puts on gloves.
- ❏ 6. Removes dental bridgework.
- ❏ 7. Wets brush and puts a small amount of toothpaste on brush.
- ❏ 8. Gently brushes teeth, including tongue and all surfaces of teeth.
- ❏ 9. Rinses mouth and allows client to spit.
- ❏ 10. Wipes client's mouth and removes towel.
- ❏ 11. Replaces dental bridgework. Applies

Name: _____   137

moisturizer to lips.

☐ 12. Disposes of water, washes and stores equipment. Removes gloves. Returns bed to lowest position.

☐ 13. Washes hands.

☐ 14. Documents procedure and any observations.

Comments:

Performing mouth care for the unconscious client

✓ **Procedure Steps**

☐ 1. Washes hands.

☐ 2. Explains procedure to client.

☐ 3. Provides privacy.

☐ 4. Adjusts the bed to a comfortable working height, if possible. Locks bed wheels.

☐ 5. Puts on gloves.

☐ 6. Turns client's head and places a towel under cheek and chin. Places basin next to cheek and chin.

☐ 7. Swabs mouth completely until clean with mouthwash-soaked swab.

☐ 8. Swabs again with lemon glycerine swab if ordered.

☐ 9. Removes towel and basin. Applies moisturizer to lips.

☐ 10. Washes and stores supplies. Removes gloves. Returns bed to lowest position.

☐ 11. Washes hands.

☐ 12. Documents procedure and any observations.

Comments:

Flossing teeth

✓ **Procedure Steps**

☐ 1. Washes hands.

☐ 2. Explains procedure to client.

☐ 3. Provides privacy.

☐ 4. Adjusts the bed to a comfortable working height, if possible. Locks bed wheels.

☐ 5. Puts on gloves.

☐ 6. Wraps floss around fingers.

☐ 7. Flosses teeth, starting with back and moving to gum line.

☐ 8. Uses clean area of floss after every two or three teeth.

☐ 9. Offers water periodically and offers a towel when done.

☐ 10. Washes and stores supplies. Removes gloves. Returns bed to lowest position.

☐ 11. Washes hands.

☐ 12. Documents procedure and any observations.

Comments:

Assisting with denture care

✓ **Procedure Steps**

☐ 1. Washes hands.

☐ 2. Explains procedure to client.

☐ 3. Provides privacy.

☐ 4. Lines sink or basin with towel and fills with water.

☐ 5. Puts on gloves.

☐ 6. Removes lower denture properly if client is unable.

☐ 7. Removes upper denture properly.

☐ 8. Applies denture cleanser to toothbrush and brushes under warm water.

☐ 9. Rinses denture cup and places dentures in it.

Name: _____

❏ 10. If client prefers, soaks dentures in solution.

❏ 11. Stores dentures in water or solution.

❏ 12. Offers client a swab or mouthwash to cleanse the mouth.

❏ 13. Washes and stores supplies. Removes gloves.

❏ 14. Washes hands.

❏ 15. Documents procedure and any observations.

Comments:

Reinserting dentures

✓ **Procedure Steps**

❏ 1. Washes hands.

❏ 2. Explains procedure to client.

❏ 3. Provides privacy.

❏ 4. Positions client in upright position.

❏ 5. Puts on gloves.

❏ 6. Applies denture cream.

❏ 7. Inserts upper denture at an angle, pressing it firmly onto upper gum line.

❏ 8. Inserts lower denture, pressing it firmly onto the lower gum line.

❏ 9. Offers client face towel.

❏ 10. Washes and stores supplies. Removes gloves.

❏ 11. Washes hands.

❏ 12. Documents procedure and any observations.

Comments:

Assisting clients in using a bedpan

✓ **Procedure Steps**

❏ 1. Washes hands.

❏ 2. Explains procedure to client.

❏ 3. Provides privacy.

❏ 4. Adjusts the bed to a comfortable working height, if possible. Locks bed wheels. Lowers head of bed.

❏ 5. Puts on gloves.

❏ 6. Warms outside of bedpan with warm water. Dusts it with talcum powder.

❏ 7. Covers client with bath blanket. Places a protective sheet under client properly, rolling client toward self. Rolls client onto back when done.

❏ 8. Asks client to remove undergarments or assists client to do so.

❏ 9. Slides bedpan under hips, helping client if necessary. Raise head of bed after placing bedpan.

❏ 10. Checks bedpan position, ensuring blanket is covering client. Provides client with supplies and leaves room until client calls.

❏ 11. If client is unable, cleans the perineum properly.

❏ 12. Discards soiled supplies properly. Dries perineal area. Removes gloves.

❏ 13. Puts on new gloves properly.

❏ 14. Offers washcloth and soap to client to wash hands. Covers client and helps put on undergarments.

❏ 15. Empties bedpan into toilet. Removes gloves. Washes hands. Puts on new gloves.

❏ 16. Rinses bedpan with cold water and empties. Cleans bedpan with hot, soapy water.

❏ 17. Removes and discards gloves.

❏ 18. Washes hands.

Name: _____

☐ 19. Documents procedure and any observations.

Comments:

Assisting clients in using a urinal

✓ **Procedure Steps**

☐ 1. Washes hands.
☐ 2. Explains procedure to client.
☐ 3. Provides privacy.
☐ 4. Adjusts the bed to a comfortable working height, if possible. Locks bed wheels.
☐ 5. Puts on gloves.
☐ 6. Places protective pad under buttocks and hips.
☐ 7. Hands urinal to client or places it if client is unable. Replaces covers.
☐ 8. Leaves room, giving client a bell.
☐ 9. Removes urinal when client is finished. Follows proper procedure if specimen is needed.
☐ 10. Discards urine and rinses urinal.
☐ 11. Removes gloves and discards them. Washes hands.
☐ 12. Gives client washcloth, soap, and water to wash his hands.
☐ 13. After discarding supplies, washes hands again. Removes gloves. Returns bed to lowest position.
☐ 14. Documents procedure and any observations.

Comments:

Assisting clients in using a portable commode or the toilet

✓ **Procedure Steps**

☐ 1. Washes hands.
☐ 2. Explains procedure to client.
☐ 3. Provides privacy.
☐ 4. Adjusts the bed to a comfortable working height, if possible. Locks bed wheels.
☐ 5. Puts on gloves.
☐ 6. Helps client to bathroom or commode.
☐ 7. Leaves room or area, giving client a bell to call.
☐ 8. Returns when client is done. Cleans perineal area if assistance is needed.
☐ 9. Helps client up and ensures client's hands are washed.
☐ 10. Removes waste container and empties into toilet.
☐ 11. Cleans container, rinsing first with cold water, then hot.
☐ 12. Removes gloves and discards them.
☐ 13. Washes hands.
☐ 14. Documents procedure and any observations.

Comments:

14

Core Healthcare Skills

Taking and recording an oral temperature

✓ **Procedure Steps**

☐ 1. Washes hands.

- [ ] 2. Explains procedure to client.
- [ ] 3. Provides privacy.

Using a mercury-free thermometer or glass thermometer:

- [ ] 4. Holds thermometer by stem.
- [ ] 5. Shakes thermometer down to below the lowest number.
- [ ] 6. Puts on disposable sheath, if available. Inserts bulb end of oral thermometer into client's mouth, under tongue and to one side.
- [ ] 7. Instructs client on how to hold thermometer in mouth.
- [ ] 8. Removes thermometer after at least three minutes. Wipes with tissue from stem to bulb or removes sheath. Disposes of tissue or sheath.
- [ ] 9. Reads temperature. Documents temperature, date, time and method used.
- [ ] 10. Rinses and dries thermometer and stores properly.

Using a digital thermometer:

- [ ] 4. Puts on disposable sheath.
- [ ] 5. Turns on thermometer and waits until "ready" sign appears.
- [ ] 6. Inserts end of digital thermometer into client's mouth, under tongue and to one side.
- [ ] 7. Removes thermometer after it blinks or beeps.
- [ ] 8. Reads temperature on display screen. Documents temperature, date, time and method used.
- [ ] 9. Removes and disposes of sheath with a tissue.
- [ ] 10. Stores thermometer.

Using an electronic thermometer:

- [ ] 4. Removes probe from base unit and puts on probe cover.
- [ ] 5. Inserts end of electronic thermometer into client's mouth, under tongue and to one side.
- [ ] 6. Removes after tone or light signals temperature has been read.
- [ ] 7. Reads temperature on display screen.
- [ ] 8. Removes the probe. Presses the eject button to discard the cover.
- [ ] 9. Documents temperature, date, time and method used.
- [ ] 10. Returns probe to holder.

Final step:

- [ ] 11. Washes hands.

Comments:

Taking and recording a rectal temperature

✓ **Procedure Steps**

- [ ] 1. Washes hands.
- [ ] 2. Explains procedure to client.
- [ ] 3. Provides privacy.
- [ ] 4. Assists client to side-lying position.
- [ ] 5. Folds back linens to only expose rectal area.
- [ ] 6. Puts on gloves.
- [ ] 7. Mercury-free or glass thermometer: Holds thermometer by stem.

Digital thermometer: Applies probe cover.

- [ ] 8. Mercury-free or glass thermometer: Shakes thermometer down to below the lowest number.
- [ ] 9. Applies a small amount of lubricant to tip or bulb or probe cover.
- [ ] 10. Gently inserts thermometer into rectum one inch. Replaces sheet over buttocks. Holds onto thermometer at all times while taking temperature.

Name: _____

141

- ❑ 11. Removes thermometer after three minutes (for a mercury-free or glass thermometer) or when it blinks or beeps (for a digital thermometer).
- ❑ 12. Wipes thermometer with tissue from stem to bulb or removes sheath.
- ❑ 13. Reads temperature. Documents temperature, date, time and method used.
- ❑ 14. Cleans and stores thermometer.
- ❑ 15. Removes and discards gloves.
- ❑ 16. Washes hands.

Comments:

Taking and recording a tympanic temperature

✓ **Procedure Steps**

- ❑ 1. Washes hands.
- ❑ 2. Explains procedure to client.
- ❑ 3. Provides privacy.
- ❑ 4. Places disposable sheath over end of thermometer.
- ❑ 5. Positions client's head properly and pulls up and back on the outside edge of the ear.
- ❑ 6. Inserts covered probe and presses the button.
- ❑ 7. Removes thermometer after one second or after it beeps.
- ❑ 8. Reads temperature. Documents temperature, date, time and method used.
- ❑ 9. Discards sheath and stores thermometer properly.
- ❑ 10. Washes hands.

Comments:

Taking and recording an axillary temperature

✓ **Procedure Steps**

- ❑ 1. Washes hands.
- ❑ 2. Explains procedure to client.
- ❑ 3. Provides privacy.
- ❑ 4. Adjusts client's clothing as necessary and makes sure axilla is dry.
- ❑ 5. Places thermometer under arm, holding it in place with the arm close against the side for eight to ten minutes.
- ❑ 6. Reads temperature. Documents temperature, date, time and method used.
- ❑ 7. Cleans and stores thermometer properly.
- ❑ 8. Washes hands.

Comments:

Taking and recording apical pulse

✓ **Procedure Steps**

- ❑ 1. Washes hands.
- ❑ 2. Explains procedure to client.
- ❑ 3. Provides privacy.
- ❑ 4. Fits earpieces of stethoscope snugly in ears and places metal diaphragm on left side of chest, just below the nipple.
- ❑ 5. Counts heartbeats for one minute.
- ❑ 6. Counts client's respirations with stethoscope still in place.
- ❑ 7. Documents pulse rate, date, time, and method used. Notes any irregularities in rhythm.
- ❑ 8. Stores stethoscope.
- ❑ 9. Washes hands.

Comments:

Taking and recording radial pulse, and counting and recording respirations

✓ **Procedure Steps**

☐ 1. Washes hands.

☐ 2. Explains procedure to client.

☐ 3. Provides privacy.

☐ 4. Places fingertips on the thumb side of client's wrist to locate pulse.

☐ 5. Counts beats for one full minute.

☐ 6. Keeping fingertips on client's wrist, counts respirations for one full minute.

☐ 7. Documents pulse rate, date, time, and method used Documents respiratory rate and the pattern or character of breathing.

☐ 8. Washes hands.

Comments:

Taking and recording blood pressure (two-step method)

✓ **Procedure Steps**

☐ 1. Washes hands.

☐ 2. Explains procedure to client.

☐ 3. Provides privacy.

☐ 4. Asks client to roll up sleeve. Positions client's arm with palm up. The arm should be level with the heart.

☐ 5. With the valve open, squeezes the cuff to make sure it is completely deflated.

☐ 6. Places blood pressure cuff snugly on client's upper arm, with the center of the cuff placed over the brachial artery.

☐ 7. Locates the radial (wrist) pulse with fingertips.

☐ 8. Closes the valve (clockwise) until it stops. Inflates cuff, watching gauge.

☐ 9. Stops inflating cuff when pulse is no longer felt. Notes the reading.

☐ 10. Opens the valve to deflate cuff completely.

☐ 11. Writes down the systolic reading.

☐ 12. Wipes diaphragm and earpieces of stethoscope with alcohol wipes.

☐ 13. Locates brachial pulse with fingertips.

☐ 14. Places earpieces of stethoscope in ears and places diaphragm of stethoscope over brachial artery.

☐ 15. Closes the valve (clockwise) until it stops. Does not tighten it.

☐ 16. Inflates cuff to 30 mm Hg above the estimated systolic pressure.

☐ 17. Opens the valve slightly with thumb and index finger. Deflates cuff slowly.

☐ 18. Watches gauge and listens for sound of pulse.

☐ 19. Remembers the reading at which the first clear pulse sound is heard. This is the systolic pressure.

☐ 20. Continues listening for a change or muffling of pulse sound. The point of a change or the point the sound disappears is the diastolic pressure. Remembers this reading.

☐ 21. Opens the valve to deflate cuff completely. Removes cuff.

☐ 22. Documents both systolic and diastolic pressures. Notes which arm was used.

☐ 23. Cleans stethoscope. Stores equipment.

☐ 24. Washes hands.

Comments:

Name: _____

Measuring and recording the weight of a client

✓ **Procedure Steps**

☐ 1. Washes hands.

☐ 2. Explains procedure to client.

☐ 3. Provides privacy.

☐ 4. Sets scale on hard floor surface and makes sure it reads zero.

☐ 5. Assists client to the scale as necessary.

☐ 6. Instructs client to step on scale, assisting as necessary. Makes sure client is not holding, touching, or leaning against anything.

☐ 7. Reads the weight.

☐ 8. Instructs client to step off the scale, and assists client back to a comfortable position.

☐ 9. Documents the weight.

☐ 10. Stores the scale.

☐ 11. Washes hands.

Comments:

Measuring and recording the height of a client

✓ **Procedure Steps**

☐ 1. Washes hands.

☐ 2. Explains procedure to client.

☐ 3. Provides privacy.

☐ 4. Positions client in bed, flat on the back, with arms and legs at sides. Makes sure bed sheet is smooth underneath client.

☐ 5. Makes a small pencil mark at the top of client's head and at client's heel.

☐ 6. Measures distance between the two marks with a tape measure.

☐ 7. Documents client's height.

☐ 8. Stores equipment.

☐ 9. Washes hands.

For clients who can get out of bed:

☐ 1. Washes hands.

☐ 2. Explains procedure to client.

☐ 3. Provides privacy.

☐ 4. Instructs client to remove shoes and stand with his back against a wall and arms at his sides.

☐ 5. Makes a small pencil mark on the wall even with the top of the client's head.

☐ 6. Instructs client to step away. Measures the distance between the pencil mark and the wall.

☐ 7. Documents height.

☐ 8. Stores equipment.

☐ 9. Washes hands.

Comments:

Collecting a sputum specimen

✓ **Procedure Steps**

☐ 1. Washes hands.

☐ 2. Explains procedure to client.

☐ 3. Provides privacy.

☐ 4. Puts on mask and gloves.

☐ 5. Gives client tissues to cover the mouth. Instructs client to cough deeply and spit the sputum into the specimen container.

☐ 6. Covers container tightly, and wipes any sputum off the outside of the container. Puts container in plastic bag, and seals it.

☐ 7. Removes gloves and mask.

☐ 8. Washes hands.

Name: _____

☐ 9. Documents the procedure and any observations.

Comments:

Collecting a stool specimen

✓ **Procedure Steps**

☐ 1. Washes hands.

☐ 2. Explains procedure to client.

☐ 3. Provides privacy.

☐ 4. Puts on gloves.

☐ 5. Asks client not to urinate at the same time as moving bowels and not to put toilet paper in with the sample. Provides plastic bag to discard toilet paper separately.

☐ 6. Fits hat to toilet or provides client with bedpan. Leaves the room and asks the client to call when he is finished.

☐ 7. Assists as necessary with perineal care. Helps client wash hands, and makes client comfortable. Removes gloves.

☐ 8. Washes hands again.

☐ 9. Puts on clean gloves.

☐ 10. Uses tongue blades to take about two tablespoons of stool and puts it in container without touching the inside. Covers container tightly.

☐ 11. Disposes of tongue blades properly. Empties bedpan or container into toilet. Cleans and stores equipment properly.

☐ 12. Stores the specimen properly.

☐ 13. Removes gloves.

☐ 14. Washes hands.

☐ 15. Documents procedure and any observations.

Comments:

Collecting a routine urine specimen

✓ **Procedure Steps**

☐ 1. Washes hands.

☐ 2. Explains procedure to client.

☐ 3. Provides privacy.

☐ 4. Puts on gloves.

☐ 5. Assists client to bathroom or commode, or offers bedpan or urinal.

☐ 6. Has client void. Asks client not to put toilet paper in with the sample. Provide a plastic bag to discard toilet paper separately.

☐ 7. Assists as necessary with perineal care. Helps client wash his or her hands. Makes client comfortable.

☐ 8. Takes bedpan, urinal, or commode pail to the bathroom.

☐ 9. Pours urine into specimen container, making it at least half full.

☐ 10. Covers container with lid. Wipes off the outside with a paper towel.

☐ 11. Places the container in a plastic bag.

☐ 12. Discards extra urine. Rinses and cleans equipment, and stores it.

☐ 13. Removes and disposes of gloves.

☐ 14. Completes label for container.

☐ 15. Washes hands.

☐ 16. Documents procedure and any observations.

Comments:

Name: _____

Collecting a clean catch (mid-stream) urine specimen

✓ Procedure Steps

- [ ] 1. Washes hands.
- [ ] 2. Explains procedure to client.
- [ ] 3. Provides privacy.
- [ ] 4. Puts on gloves.
- [ ] 5. Opens specimen kit.
- [ ] 6. Cleans the area around the urethra.
- [ ] 7. Asks client to urinate into the bedpan, urinal, or toilet, and to stop before urination is complete.
- [ ] 8. Places container under the urine stream and instructs client to start urinating again until container is at least half full.
- [ ] 9. Covers urine container and wipes off outside with paper towel.
- [ ] 10. Discards extra urine. Rinses and cleans equipment, and stores it.
- [ ] 11. Removes gloves and washes hands. Assists client to wash hands.
- [ ] 12. Completes label for container.
- [ ] 13. Washes hands again.
- [ ] 14. Documents procedure and any observations.

Comments:

Collecting a 24-hour urine specimen

✓ Procedure Steps

- [ ] 1. Washes hands.
- [ ] 2. Explains procedure to client.
- [ ] 3. Provides privacy.
- [ ] 4. Instructs client to completely empty the bladder. Discards urine and notes the exact time.
- [ ] 5. Labels container.
- [ ] 6. Puts on gloves each time client voids.
- [ ] 7. Pours urine into container using the funnel as needed.
- [ ] 8. Assists client to wash hands after each voiding.
- [ ] 9. Instructs family to save all urine and store properly after each voiding.
- [ ] 10. Cleans equipment after each voiding.
- [ ] 11. Removes gloves.
- [ ] 12. Washes hands.
- [ ] 13. Documents procedure and any observations.

Comments:

Measuring and recording input and output

✓ Procedure Steps

- [ ] 1. Washes hands.
- [ ] 2. Explains procedure to client.
- [ ] 3. Provides privacy.
- [ ] 4. Measures amount of fluid client is served and notes on paper, not visit notes.
- [ ] 5. Measures leftover fluids and notes on paper, not visit notes.
- [ ] 6. Subtracts amount left over from amount served. Converts to cubic centimeters.
- [ ] 7. Documents amount of fluids consumed (in cc), time, and what fluid was taken in visit notes.

For measuring the client's output:

- [ ] 1. Washes hands.
- [ ] 2. Explains procedure to client.
- [ ] 3. Provides privacy.
- [ ] 4. Puts on gloves.

Name: _____

- [ ] 5. Asks client not to urinate at same time as moving bowels. Asks client to put used toilet paper in plastic bag, not with the sample.
- [ ] 6. Makes client comfortable and leaves room if assistance is not needed.
- [ ] 7. Assists client with handwashing as necessary.
- [ ] 8. Pours urine into measuring container and notes the amount on paper.
- [ ] 9. Discards urine and toilet paper properly. Washes and stores equipment properly.
- [ ] 10. Removes gloves.
- [ ] 11. Washes hands.
- [ ] 12. Documents the time, amount (in cc), and color of urine.

Comments:

Observing, reporting, and documenting client's emesis

✓ **Procedure Steps**

- [ ] 1. Puts on gloves.
- [ ] 2. Provides a basin and removes it when vomiting has stopped.
- [ ] 3. Removes soiled linens or clothes and replaces with fresh ones.
- [ ] 4. Measures and notes amount of vomitus, if monitoring client's I&O.
- [ ] 5. Discards vomit in toilet and washes and stores basin properly.
- [ ] 6. Removes gloves.
- [ ] 7. Washes hands.
- [ ] 8. Puts on fresh gloves.
- [ ] 9. Provides comfort to client.
- [ ] 10. Launders soiled linens and clothes in hot water.
- [ ] 11. Removes gloves.
- [ ] 12. Washes hands again.
- [ ] 13. Documents time, amount, color, and consistency of vomitus. Observes for blood.
- [ ] 14. Reports to supervisor immediately.

Comments:

Providing catheter care

✓ **Procedure Steps**

- [ ] 1. Washes hands.
- [ ] 2. Explains procedure to client.
- [ ] 3. Provides privacy.
- [ ] 4. Adjusts the bed to a comfortable working height, if possible. Lowers head of bed and positions client lying flat on back. Raises side rail farthest from self.
- [ ] 5. Removes or folds back top bedding, keeping client covered with bath blanket.
- [ ] 6. Makes sure water temperature is 105° to 109° F.
- [ ] 7. Puts on gloves.
- [ ] 8. Places clean protective pad under buttocks.
- [ ] 9. Exposes only the area necessary to clean the catheter.
- [ ] 10. Places towel or pad under catheter tubing before washing.
- [ ] 11. Holding catheter near meatus, cleans at least four inches of catheter. Moves in only one direction, away from meatus. Uses a clean area of the cloth for each stroke.
- [ ] 12. Rinses at least four inches of catheter nearest meatus.
- [ ] 13. Empties water into toilet. Disposes of linen in proper containers.

Name: _____

- ☐ 14. Removes and disposes of gloves. Returns bed to lowest position.
- ☐ 15. Washes hands.
- ☐ 16. Helps client dress. Arranges covers. Checks that catheter tubing is free from kinks and twists and that it is securely taped to the leg.
- ☐ 17. Washes hands again.
- ☐ 18. Documents procedure and any observations.

Comments:

Emptying the catheter drainage bag

✓ **Procedure Steps**

- ☐ 1. Washes hands.
- ☐ 2. Explains procedure to client.
- ☐ 3. Puts on gloves.
- ☐ 4. Places measuring container on paper towel on floor.
- ☐ 5. Opens drain or spout on bag so urine flows into measuring container.
- ☐ 6. Closes spout and cleans it. Replaces drain in its holder on the bag.
- ☐ 7. Notes amount and appearance of urine and empties it into toilet.
- ☐ 8. Cleans and stores measuring container properly.
- ☐ 9. Removes gloves.
- ☐ 10. Washes hands.
- ☐ 11. Documents procedure and any observations.

Comments:

Applying a condom catheter

✓ **Procedure Steps**

- ☐ 1. Washes hands.
- ☐ 2. Explains procedure to client.
- ☐ 3. Provides privacy.
- ☐ 4. Adjusts the bed to a comfortable working height, if possible. Lowers head of bed and positions client lying flat on back. Raises side rail farthest from self.
- ☐ 5. Removes or folds back bedding, keeping client covered with bath blanket.
- ☐ 6. Puts on gloves.
- ☐ 7. Adjusts bath blanket to only expose genital area.
- ☐ 8. Removes condom catheter if one if in place.
- ☐ 9. Assists as necessary with perineal care.
- ☐ 10. Attaches collection bag to leg.
- ☐ 11. Places condom on penis and rolls towards base of penis, leaving space between drainage tip and glans of penis to prevent irritation.
- ☐ 12. Secure condom to penis.
- ☐ 13. Connects catheter tip to drainage tubing. Makes sure tubing is not twisted or kinked.
- ☐ 14. Discards used supplies in plastic bag.
- ☐ 15. Removes and disposes of gloves. Returns bed to its lowest position.
- ☐ 16. Washes hands.
- ☐ 17. Removes bath blanket and store it. Makes client comfortable.
- ☐ 18. Documents procedure and any observations.

Comments:

Name: _____

Preparing and applying warm compresses

✓ **Procedure Steps**

☐ 1. Washes hands.

☐ 2. Explains procedure to client.

☐ 3. Provides privacy.

☐ 4. Fills basin with hot water (105° to 115°F).

☐ 5. Soaks wash cloth, wrings it out, and applies to area needing compress. Covers with plastic wrap and towel.

☐ 6. Notes the time. Checks area every five minutes. Changes compress if cooling occurs.

☐ 7. Removes compress after 20 minutes, or if area is red, numb, or client complains of pain or discomfort.

☐ 8. Discards water. Cleans and stores basin and other supplies properly. Puts laundry in hamper, and discards plastic wrap.

☐ 9. Washes hands.

☐ 10. Documents time, length, and site of procedure, and any observations.

Comments:

Administering warm soaks

✓ **Procedure Steps**

☐ 1. Washes hands.

☐ 2. Explains procedure to client.

☐ 3. Provides privacy.

☐ 4. Fill the basin or tub half full of warm water (105° to 110°F).

☐ 5. Immerses body part in water properly, padding the edge of the basin as necessary. Covers client for extra warmth if needed.

☐ 6. Checks water temperature every five minutes, adding hot water as needed.

☐ 7. Observes area for redness and discontinues soak if client complains of pain or discomfort.

☐ 8. Soaks for 15 to 20 minutes or as ordered in the care plan.

☐ 9. Removes basin or helps client out of the tub. Dries the client.

☐ 10. Drains tub or discards water in basin. Cleans and stores basin and other supplies. Puts laundry in hamper.

☐ 11. Washes hands.

☐ 12. Documents time, length, and site of procedure, and any observations. Reports client's response and observations about skin.

Comments:

Using a hot water bottle

✓ **Procedure Steps**

☐ 1. Washes hands.

☐ 2. Explains procedure to client.

☐ 3. Provides privacy.

☐ 4. Fills bottle halfway with warm water (105° to 110°F), presses out excess air, and seals bottle.

☐ 5. Dries the bottle and checks for leaks. Covers bottle with cloth or towel.

☐ 6. Applies bottle to the area. Checks skin every five minutes for redness or pain. Adds cold water to bottle if skin is red or client complains of pain.

☐ 7. Removes bottle after 20 minutes or as ordered in the care plan.

☐ 8. Empties bottle, and washes and stores supplies.

☐ 9. Washes hands.

☐ 10. Documents time, length, and site of procedure, and any observations.

Name: _____

Comments:

Assisting with a sitz bath

✓ **Procedure Steps**

- ☐ 1. Washes hands.
- ☐ 2. Explains procedure to client.
- ☐ 3. Provides privacy.
- ☐ 4. Puts on gloves.
- ☐ 5. Fills sitz bath two-thirds full with hot water (100°F-104°F or 105°F-110°F, depending on the reason for the bath).
- ☐ 6. Places sitz bath on toilet seat and helps client undress and sit down on sitz bath.
- ☐ 7. Leaves the room and checks on client every five minutes for weakness or dizziness. Stays with client who is unsteady.
- ☐ 8. Assists client out of sitz bath after 20 minutes. Provides towels and helps with dressing as needed.
- ☐ 9. Cleans and stores supplies properly.
- ☐ 10. Washes hands.
- ☐ 11. Documents procedure, including the time started and ended, the client's response, and the water temperature

Comments:

Applying ice packs

✓ **Procedure Steps**

- ☐ 1. Washes hands.
- ☐ 2. Explains procedure to client.
- ☐ 3. Provides privacy.
- ☐ 4. Fills plastic bag with ice and removes excess air. Covers bag with towel.
- ☐ 5. Applies bag to the area as ordered. Uses another towel to cover bag if it is too cold.
- ☐ 6. Notes the time and checks the area after ten minutes for blisters, pale, white, or gray skin. Stops treatment if client complains of numbness or pain.
- ☐ 7. Removes ice after 20 minutes or as ordered in the care plan. Returns ice bag to freezer.
- ☐ 8. Washes hands.
- ☐ 9. Document the time, length, and site of procedure. Report the client's response and any of your observations about the skin.

Comments:

Applying cold compresses

✓ **Procedure Steps**

- ☐ 1. Washes hands.
- ☐ 2. Explains procedure to client.
- ☐ 3. Provides privacy.
- ☐ 4. Positions client, rinses washcloth in basin, and wrings out washcloth.
- ☐ 5. Covers the area with sheet or towel and applies cold washcloth to the area. Changes washcloths to keep area cold.
- ☐ 6. Checks the area after five minutes for blisters, pale, white, or gray skin. Stops treatment if client complains of numbness or pain.
- ☐ 7. Removes compresses after 20 minutes or as ordered in the care plan. Gives client towels as needed to dry the area.
- ☐ 8. Cleans and stores basin properly.

- ❏ 9. Washes hands.
- ❏ 10. Documents the time, length, and site of procedure. Reports the client's response and any observations about the skin.

Comments:

Changing a dry dressing using non-sterile technique

✓ **Procedure Steps**

- ❏ 1. Washes hands.
- ❏ 2. Explains procedure to client.
- ❏ 3. Provides privacy.
- ❏ 4. Cuts pieces of tape long enough to secure the dressing. Opens gauze package without touching the gauze.
- ❏ 5. Puts on gloves.
- ❏ 6. Removes soiled dressing gently, observing dressing for odor or drainage. Notes color of the wound. Disposes of used dressing in the waste bag. Removes and discards gloves in the waste bag.
- ❏ 7. Puts on new gloves.
- ❏ 8. Applies clean gauze to wound. Tapes gauze in place.
- ❏ 9. Removes and discards gloves in the waste bag.
- ❏ 10. Washes hands.
- ❏ 11. Documents procedure and any observations.

Comments:

Applying anti-embolic hose

✓ **Procedure Steps**

- ❏ 1. Washes hands.
- ❏ 2. Explains procedure to client.
- ❏ 3. Provides privacy.
- ❏ 4. With client lying down, removes his or her socks, shoes, or slippers, and exposes one leg.
- ❏ 5. Turns stocking inside-out at least to heel area
- ❏ 6. Gently places the foot of the stocking over toes, foot, and heel.
- ❏ 7. Gently pulls top of stocking over foot, heel, and leg.
- ❏ 8. Makes sure that there are no twists and wrinkles in the stocking after it is applied.
- ❏ 9. Repeats for the other leg.
- ❏ 10. Washes hands.
- ❏ 11. Documents procedure and any observations.

Comments:

Caring for an ostomy

✓ **Procedure Steps**

- ❏ 1. Washes hands.
- ❏ 2. Explains procedure to client.
- ❏ 3. Provides privacy.
- ❏ 4. Adjusts the bed to a comfortable working height, if possible.
- ❏ 5. Places bed protector under client. Covers client with a bath blanket and only exposes the ostomy site.
- ❏ 6. Puts on gloves.
- ❏ 7. Removes ostomy bag carefully. Notes color, odor, consistency, and amount of stool in the bag.
- ❏ 8. Wipes area around the stoma with toilet paper. Discards paper in plastic bag.

Name: _____

- ❏ 9. Washes area around the stoma using a washcloth and warm soapy water. Pats dry with another towel. Applies cream if ordered.
- ❏ 10. Places the clean ostomy appliance on client, following instructions. Makes sure the bottom of the bag is clamped.
- ❏ 11. Removes disposable bed protector and discards.
- ❏ 12. Removes gloves. Makes the client comfortable. Puts on fresh gloves to change linens if necessary. Covers client and removes bath blanket and towel.
- ❏ 13. Places soiled linens in appropriate containers. Removes gloves.
- ❏ 14. Puts on new gloves. Cleans bedpan. Stores bedpan and supplies.
- ❏ 15. Removes and disposes of gloves. Returns bed to lowest level.
- ❏ 16. Washes hands.
- ❏ 17. Documents procedure and any observations.

Comments:

15

Rehabilitation and Restorative Care

Assisting with passive range of motion (PROM) exercises

✓ Procedure Steps

- ❏ 1. Washes hands.
- ❏ 2. Explains procedure to client.
- ❏ 3. Provides privacy.
- ❏ 4. Adjusts the bed to a comfortable working height, if possible. Locks bed wheels.
- ❏ 5. Positions client in supine position.

Shoulder:
Performs the following movements properly, supporting the client's arm at the elbow and wrist by placing one hand above the elbow and the other hand around the wrist:

- ❏ 1. Forward flexion
- ❏ 2. Extension
- ❏ 3. Abduction
- ❏ 4. Adduction
- ❏ 5. Internal rotation
- ❏ 6. External rotation

Elbow:
Performs the following movements properly, holding the wrist with one hand, and holding the elbow with the other:

- ❏ 1. Flexion
- ❏ 2. Extension
- ❏ 3. Pronation
- ❏ 4. Supination

Wrist:
Performs the following movements properly, holding the wrist with one hand, and using the fingers of the other hand to help the joint through the motions :

- ❏ 1. Flexion
- ❏ 2. Extension
- ❏ 3. Radial flexion
- ❏ 4. Ulnar flexion

Thumb:
Performs the following movements properly:

- ❏ 1. Abduction
- ❏ 2. Adduction
- ❏ 3. Opposition
- ❏ 4. Flexion

Name: _____

- [ ] 5. Extension

    Fingers:
    Performs the following movements properly:

- [ ] 1. Flexion
- [ ] 2. Extension
- [ ] 3. Abduction
- [ ] 4. Adduction

    Hip:
    Performs the following movements properly, placing one hand under the knee and one under the ankle:

- [ ] 1. Abduction
- [ ] 2. Adduction
- [ ] 3. Internal rotation
- [ ] 4. External rotation

    Knees:
    Performs the following movements properly:

- [ ] 1. Flexion
- [ ] 2. Extension

    Ankles:
    Performs the following movements properly:

- [ ] 1. Dorsiflexion
- [ ] 2. Plantar flexion
- [ ] 3. Supination
- [ ] 4. Pronation

    Toes:
    Performs the following movements properly:

- [ ] 1. Flexion
- [ ] 2. Extension
- [ ] 3. Abduction

When all exercises are completed:

- [ ] 6. Returns client to comfortable position and covers as appropriate. Returns bed to lowest position.
- [ ] 7. Washes hands.
- [ ] 8. Documents procedure. Notes any decrease in range of motion or any pain experienced by the client. Notifies supervisor if increased stiffness or physical resistance is noted.

Comments:

Assisting with deep breathing exercises

✓ **Procedure Steps**

- [ ] 1. Washes hands.
- [ ] 2. Explains procedure to client.
- [ ] 3. Provides privacy.
- [ ] 4. Puts on mask, eye shield, and gown.
- [ ] 5. Puts on gloves.
- [ ] 6. Has client inhale deeply while sitting up.
- [ ] 7. Has client exhale completely.
- [ ] 8. Repeats exercise five to ten times.
- [ ] 9. Offers tissues if necessary.
- [ ] 10. Disposes of tissues and cleans basin.
- [ ] 11. Removes gloves, eye shield, mask, and gown properly.
- [ ] 12. Washes hands.
- [ ] 13. Puts on new gloves properly.
- [ ] 14. Provides mouth care.
- [ ] 15. Removes gloves and washes hands.
- [ ] 16. Documents procedure and any observations.

Comments:

Name: _____

16

Medications and Technology in Home Care

Assisting in changing clothes for a client who has an IV

✓ **Procedure Steps**

- ☐ 1. Washes hands.
- ☐ 2. Explains procedure to client.
- ☐ 3. Provides privacy.
- ☐ 4. Adjusts bed to lowest position, if possible, and helps client sit up at the edge of the bed.
- ☐ 5. Helps client remove the arm without the IV from the clothing.
- ☐ 6. Helps client gather clothing on arm with IV site, lift clothing over IV site, and move it up the tubing towards the IV bag.
- ☐ 7. Lifts IV bag off the pole, keeping it higher than the IV site, slides clothing over IV bag, and replaces IV bag on the pole.
- ☐ 8. Sets used clothing aside and gathers the sleeve of the clean clothing.
- ☐ 9. Lifts IV bag off the pole again, keeping it higher than the IV site, slides clean clothing over IV bag onto the client's arm, and replaces IV bag on the pole.
- ☐ 10. Moves clean clothing over tubing and IV site and onto the client's arm.
- ☐ 11. Assists client with putting other arm into clothing.
- ☐ 12. Checks the IV, the tubing, and dressing for proper placement.
- ☐ 13. Assists client with changing the rest of the clothing.
- ☐ 14. Places soiled laundry in laundry basket, and adjusts bed, if necessary.
- ☐ 15. Washes hands.
- ☐ 16. Documents procedure and any observations.

Comments:

19

New Mothers, Infants and Children

Picking up and holding a baby

✓ **Procedure Steps**

- ☐ 1. Washes hands.
- ☐ 2. Supports the head at all times when lifting or holding a baby. With the other hand, supports the baby's back and bottom.
- ☐ 3. Performs cradle hold properly.
- ☐ 4. Performs football hold properly.
- ☐ 5. Performs upright hold properly.

Comments:

Sterilizing bottles

✓ **Procedure Steps**

- ☐ 1. Washes hands.
- ☐ 2. Boils water and puts equipment in.
- ☐ 3. Re-boils water for five minutes.
- ☐ 4. Removes equipment and discards water. Stores when dry.

Comments:

Name: _____

Assisting with bottle feeding

✓ **Procedure Steps**

- [ ] 1. Washes hands.
- [ ] 2. Prepares bottle.
- [ ] 3. Sits and holds baby properly.
- [ ] 4. Inserts bottle nipple, and ensures that baby's head is higher than body.
- [ ] 5. Talks or sings to baby during feeding.
- [ ] 6. Burps baby, changes diaper, and puts baby down.
- [ ] 7. Washes hands.
- [ ] 8. Documents procedure and any observations.
- [ ] 9. Washes and sterilizes bottle.

Comments:

Burping a baby

✓ **Procedure Steps**

- [ ] 1. Washes hands.
- [ ] 2. Assembles correct equipment.
- [ ] 3. Picks baby up, using either of the two safe positions.
- [ ] 4. Pats back gently until baby burps.
- [ ] 5. Returns baby to safe position.

Comments:

Giving an infant sponge bath

✓ **Procedure Steps**

- [ ] 1. Washes hands.
- [ ] 2. Puts on gloves.
- [ ] 3. Fills basin and tests temperature.
- [ ] 4. Holds baby in football hold and washes eyes, then rest of face, using no soap.
- [ ] 5. Holds baby in football hold and washes hair.
- [ ] 6. Lays baby down, keeping one hand on baby.
- [ ] 7. Undresses upper body and washes it. Dries and covers the baby.
- [ ] 8. Undresses lower body, washes and dries it.
- [ ] 9. Washes perineal area properly.
- [ ] 10. Washes bottom and dries completely.
- [ ] 11. Applies lotion, keeping baby covered.
- [ ] 12. Diapers and dresses baby. Returns baby to safe position.
- [ ] 13. Discards water, cleans supplies, and discards gloves.
- [ ] 14. Washes hands.
- [ ] 15. Documents procedure and any observations.

Comments:

Giving an infant tub bath

✓ **Procedure Steps**

- [ ] 1. Washes hands.
- [ ] 2. Puts on gloves.
- [ ] 3. Fills basin and tests temperature.
- [ ] 4. Holds baby in football hold and washes eyes, then rest of face, using no soap.
- [ ] 5. Holds baby in football hold and washes hair.
- [ ] 6. Lays baby down, undresses, and immerses baby in basin, keeping head above water.
- [ ] 7. Uses washcloth to wash from neck down.

Name: _____

❑ 8. Removes from bath and covers immediately.

❑ 9. Applies lotion, keeping baby covered.

❑ 10. Diapers and dresses baby. Returns baby to safe position.

❑ 11. Washes hands.

❑ 12. Documents procedure and any observations.

Comments:

Changing cloth or disposable diapers

✓ **Procedure Steps**

❑ 1. Washes hands.

❑ 2. Puts on gloves.

❑ 3. Undresses baby as necessary and removes diaper.

❑ 4. Cleans perineal area.

❑ 5. Applies ointment as necessary and allows air to circulate.

❑ 6. Applies cloth or disposable diaper properly.

❑ 7. Dresses baby and returns to safe position.

❑ 8. Disposes of diaper properly.

❑ 9. Removes gloves properly.

❑ 10. Washes hands.

❑ 11. Cleans area and stores supplies.

❑ 12. Documents procedure and any observations.

Comments:

Taking an infant's axillary or tympanic temperature

✓ **Procedure Steps**

❑ 1. Washes hands.

❑ 2. Prepares thermometer.

For axillary temperature:

❑ 3. Undresses baby on one side and lays baby down.

❑ 4. Takes temperature, keeping thermometer in place for three to five minutes.

For tympanic temperature:

❑ 3. Lays baby on side.

❑ 4. Takes temperature, making sure ear is sealed.

❑ 5. Reads temperature, dresses baby, and returns to safe position.

❑ 6. Washes hands.

❑ 7. Documents temperature.

Comments:

20

Common Chronic and Acute Conditions

Providing foot care for the diabetic client

✓ **Procedure Steps**

❑ 1. Washes hands.

❑ 2. Explains procedure to client.

❑ 3. Provides privacy.

❑ 4. Puts on gloves if client has broken skin.

❑ 5. Washes feet with washcloth and soap, and rinses in warm water.

Name: _____

- ❏ 6. Pats the feet dry, wiping between the toes.
- ❏ 7. Gently rubs lotion into the feet with circular strokes.
- ❏ 8. Observes the skin for signs of dryness, irritation, etc.
- ❏ 9. Assists client with putting on socks and shoes or slippers.
- ❏ 10. Disposes of used linens properly and cleans and stores basin and supplies.
- ❏ 11. Removes gloves if worn.
- ❏ 12. Washes hands.
- ❏ 13. Documents procedure and any observations.

Comments:

21

Clean, Safe and Healthy Environments

Cleaning a bathroom

✓ **Procedure Steps**

- ❏ 1. Puts on gloves.
- ❏ 2. Wipes all surfaces with disinfectant and sponge.
- ❏ 3. Wipes toilet bowl, using different sponge.
- ❏ 4. Cleans bathtub, shower, and sink, using a different sponge.
- ❏ 5. Scrubs inside of toilet bowl with brush.
- ❏ 6. Washes floor.
- ❏ 7. Cleans mirror and all glass.
- ❏ 8. Disposes of soiled towels and waste.

- ❏ 9. Stores supplies. Removes and discards gloves.
- ❏ 10. Washes hands.
- ❏ 11. Documents procedure and any observations.

Comments:

Doing the laundry

✓ **Procedure Steps**

- ❏ 1. Sorts clothes carefully, checking pockets and garments.
- ❏ 2. Pretreats clothes as necessary.
- ❏ 3. Uses correct temperature, laundry products, and washing cycle.
- ❏ 4. Dries clothes.
- ❏ 5. Hand-washes as necessary.
- ❏ 6. Folds and hangs clean laundry. Stores clothes.

Comments:

Making an occupied bed

✓ **Procedure Steps**

- ❏ 1. Washes hands.
- ❏ 2. Explains procedure to client.
- ❏ 3. Provides privacy.
- ❏ 4. Places clean linen within reach.
- ❏ 5. Adjusts the bed to a comfortable working height, if possible. Locks bed wheels.
- ❏ 6. Puts on gloves.
- ❏ 7. Covers client and loosens top linen.
- ❏ 8. Raises side rail and rolls client to one side.

Name: _____

- [ ] 9. Loosens bottom soiled linen, mattress pad, and protector on opposite side of bed.
- [ ] 10. Rolls bottom soiled linen toward client, tucking it snugly against the client's back.
- [ ] 11. Places and tucks in clean bottom linen, finishing with no wrinkles. Makes hospital corners if necessary.
- [ ] 12. Smoothes bottom sheet out toward the client. Rolls extra material toward client and tucks it under client's body.
- [ ] 13. Places waterproof pad if using and centers it. Smoothes it out toward client, and tucks it under client's body.
- [ ] 14. Places draw sheet if using. Smoothes and tucks as with other bedding.
- [ ] 15. Assists client to turn onto clean bottom sheet towards self. Raises side rail nearest self and lowers side rail on other side of bed.
- [ ] 16. Loosens soiled linen. Rolls linen from head to the foot of bed, avoiding contact with skin or clothes. Places it in a hamper or basket.
- [ ] 17. Pulls and tucks in clean bottom linen just like other side, finishing with bottom sheet free of wrinkles.
- [ ] 18. Asks client to turn onto his or her back, keeping client covered.
- [ ] 19. Unfolds top sheet and places it over client. Slips blanket or old sheet out from underneath. Puts it in the laundry hamper.
- [ ] 20. Places a blanket over the top sheet, matching the top edges. Tucks bottom edges of top sheet and blanket under mattress, making square corners on each side. Loosens top linens over client's feet. Folds top sheet over the blanket about six inches.
- [ ] 21. Removes pillow and pillowcase. Places it in the laundry hamper. Removes gloves.
- [ ] 22. Places clean pillowcases on pillows. Places them under client's head.
- [ ] 23. Returns bed to lowest position. Carries laundry hamper to laundry area.
- [ ] 24. Washes hands.
- [ ] 25. Documents procedure and any observations.

Comments:

Making an unoccupied bed

✓ **Procedure Steps**

- [ ] 1. Washes hands.
- [ ] 2. Adjusts the bed to a comfortable working height, if possible. Locks bed wheels.
- [ ] 3. Puts on gloves.
- [ ] 4. Loosens soiled linen and rolls it from head to foot of bed. Avoids contact with skin or clothes. Places it in a hamper or basket. Removes gloves.
- [ ] 5. Remakes bed, spreading mattress pad and bottom sheet, tucking under. Makes hospital corners. Puts on mattress protector and draw sheet, smoothes, and tucks under sides of bed.
- [ ] 6. Places top sheet and blanket, centering them. Tucks under end of bed and makes hospital corners. Folds down top sheet over the blanket about six inches.
- [ ] 7. Removes pillows and pillowcases. Removes gloves. Puts on clean pillowcases. Replaces pillows.
- [ ] 8. Returns bed to its lowest position. Carries laundry hamper to laundry area.
- [ ] 9. Washes hands.
- [ ] 10. Documents procedure and any observations.

Comments:

Name: _____

23

Meal Planning, Shopping, Preparation, and Storage

Assisting a client with eating

✓ **Procedure Steps**

☐ 1. Washes hands.

☐ 2. Explains procedure to client.

☐ 3. Assist client to wash hands.

☐ 4. Ensures client is in upright sitting position.

☐ 5. Assists client to put on clothing protector, if desired.

☐ 6. Sits at client's eye level.

☐ 7. Checks temperature of food. Offers food in bite-sized pieces and alternates types of food offered. Makes sure client's mouth is empty before offering the next bite of food or sip of drink.

☐ 8. Offers drinks throughout the meal.

☐ 9. Wipes client's mouth and hands as necessary.

☐ 10. Talks with client during meal.

☐ 11. Removes clothing protector if used. Removes tray or dishes.

☐ 12. Washes hands.

☐ 13. Assists client to a comfortable position.

☐ 14. Documents procedure (including client's intake, if required) and any observations.

Comments:

Name:_____

159

Name: